## Disclaimer

This book is designed to provide accurate and authoritative information in regard to the subject matter covered. It is sold with the understanding that the publisher and author are not engaged in rendering medical, legal, or other professional advice. The information contained in this book is for educational and linguistic reference purposes only.

It is not intended as a substitute for professional medical advice, diagnosis, or treatment. Always seek the advice of a physician or other qualified health provider with any questions you may have regarding a medical condition or patient communication. Healthcare professionals should rely on their own clinical judgment and verify critical information. Communication in healthcare is complex and nuanced; this guide is a support tool and cannot cover every possible situation.

The publisher and the author assume no liability for errors or omissions, or for any consequences arising from the use of the information contained herein.

## Found a Mistake?

If you notice any errors in the writing, formatting, or printing of this book, please contact us at:

**sergio@acquirealot.com**. We'll be happy to assist you and resolve the issue as quickly as possible.

**Paperback ISBN:** 979-8-9923568-2-3

## Cover Design:

Ingrid Pilar

**Printed in the United States**

First Edition, 2025.

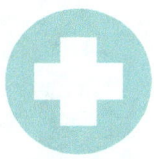

# TABLE OF CONTENTS

**Introduction** . . . . . . . . . . . . . . . . . . . . . . . . . . . . . . . . . . . . . . . . . . . 1

A Progressive 15-Minute Daily Plan to Master This Book . . . . . . . . . . 2

How to Progress Through the Book, Chapter by Chapter: . . . . . . . . 2

## Book 1

## Foundations of Medical Spanish for Healthcare Professionals

**Chapter 1: Medical Spanish for Healthcare Professionals** . . . . . . . 5

1.1 Why Medical Spanish? Meeting the Needs of Spanish-Speaking Patients. . . . . . . . . . . . . . . . . . . . . . . . . . . . . . . . . . . . . . . . . . . . . . . . 5

1.2 Key Linguistic Differences Between English and Medical Spanish . . . . . . . . . . . . . . . . . . . . . . . . . . . . . . . . . . . . . . . . . . . . . . . . 7

1.3 Pronunciation Essentials for Clear Communication. . . . . . . . . . . 12

1.4 Basic Medical Vocabulary: Core Terms and Concepts. . . . . . . . . 15

1.5 Common Grammatical Structures in Medical Contexts. . . . . . . . 17

## Book 2

## Clinical Consultation in Spanish

**Chapter 2: Essential Phrases for Initial Patient Encounters**. . . . 21

2.1 Greetings and Introductions: Formal and Informal. . . . . . . . . . . . 21

2.2 Asking for Patient Identification and Basic Information . . . . . . . 23

2.3 Establishing Rapport and Addressing Patient Comfort . . . . . . . 25

2.4 Explaining the Purpose of the Encounter . . . . . . . . . . . . . . . . . . . 27

2.5 Basic Questions About Symptoms and Well-being . . . . . . . . . . 28

2.6 Practical Exercise: Basic Questions in Spanish . . . . . . . . . . . . . . . 30

**Chapter 3: Understanding Patient History and Symptoms** . . . . 33

3.1 Asking About Past Medical History and Conditions. . . . . . . . . . . 33

3.2 Describing Pain: Location, Type, Intensity . . . . . . . . . . . . . . . . . . . 35

3.3 Asking About Allergies and Medications . . . . . . . . . . . . . . . . . . . . 38

3.4 Gathering Social History Relevant to Health. . . . . . . . . . . . . . . .40

3.5 Practical Exercise. . . . . . . . . . . . . . . . . . . . . . . . . . . . . . . . . . . . . . . .42

## Book 3

## Performing the Physical Exam in Spanish

**Chapter 4: Explaining Examination Procedures**. . . . . . . . . . . . .47

4.1 Describing Examination Steps: Inspection, Palpation,
Percussion, Auscultation. . . . . . . . . . . . . . . . . . . . . . . . . . . . . . . . . . . . .47

4.2 Giving Instructions for Patient Positioning and Cooperation. .49

4.3 Explaining the Use of Medical Instruments . . . . . . . . . . . . . . . . .49

4.4 Ensuring Patient Comfort and Addressing Concerns . . . . . . . .50

**Chapter 5: Describing Physical Examination Findings** . . . . . . . .52

5.1 General Appearance and Vital Signs. . . . . . . . . . . . . . . . . . . . . . .52

5.2 Cardiovascular Examination: Heart Sounds and Pulses . . . . . . .53

5.3 Abdominal Examination: Bowel Sounds and Palpation . . . . . . .55

5.4 Musculoskeletal Examination: Range of Motion and Strength 56

**Chapter 6: Documenting Examination Findings in Spanish** . . . 61

6.1 Common Abbreviations and Acronyms in Spanish Medical
Notes . . . . . . . . . . . . . . . . . . . . . . . . . . . . . . . . . . . . . . . . . . . . . . . . . . . . . . 61

6.2 Describing Normal and Abnormal Findings Using Precise
Terminology . . . . . . . . . . . . . . . . . . . . . . . . . . . . . . . . . . . . . . . . . . . . . . . .62

6.3 Documenting Vital Signs and Measurements. . . . . . . . . . . . . . .64

6.4 Writing Concise and Accurate Examination Reports. . . . . . . . .65

## Book 4

## Discussing Diagnosis and Treatment with Spanish-Speaking Patients

**Chapter 7: Explaining Diagnostic Tests to Patients** . . . . . . . . . . .69

7.1 Introducing the Need for Diagnostic Tests. . . . . . . . . . . . . . . . . .69

7.2 Describing Common Laboratory Tests (Blood Test, Urine
Analysis) . . . . . . . . . . . . . . . . . . . . . . . . . . . . . . . . . . . . . . . . . . . . . . . . . . . .70

7.3 Explaining Imaging Procedures (X-ray, Ultrasound, CT scan,
MRI). . . . . . . . . . . . . . . . . . . . . . . . . . . . . . . . . . . . . . . . . . . . . . . . . . . . . . . . 71

7.4 Describing Endoscopic Procedures (Colonoscopy, Gastroscopy)
. . . . . . . . . . . . . . . . . . . . . . . . . . . . . . . . . . . . . . . . . . . . . . . . . . . . . . . . . . . .73

7.5 Explaining Cardiac Tests (ECG, Echocardiogram) . . . . . . . . . . . .74

**Chapter 8: Discussing Test Results and Diagnoses** . . . . . . . . . . .79

8.1 Explaining Normal and Abnormal Test Results Clearly. . . . . . . .79

8.2 Communicating a Diagnosis with Sensitivity and Clarity...... 81

8.3 Discussing Differential Diagnoses............................83

8.4 Addressing Patient Questions and Concerns About Test Results
.......................................................................84

**Chapter 9: Explaining Treatment Options** ...................89

9.1 Introducing Different Treatment Modalities (Medication, Therapy, Surgery)...............................................89

9.2 Describing Medications: Dosage, Frequency, Route of Administration.................................................90

9.3 Explaining Surgical Procedures and Pre/Post-operative Instructions.....................................................92

9.4 Discussing Physical Therapy and Rehabilitation Plans ........93

9.5 Addressing Alternative and Complementary Therapies.......95

Book **5**

## Effective Patient Education in Spanish

**Chapter 10: Providing Instructions on Medication and Self-Care**
.................................................................... 101

10.1 Giving Clear Instructions on How to Take Medications....... 101

10.2 Explaining Potential Side Effects and What to Do...........103

10.3 Providing Guidance on Wound Care and Hygiene ..........104

10.4 Instructing Patients on Dietary Modifications and Lifestyle Changes.................................................106

10.5 Explaining the Importance of Follow-Up Appointments ....107

**Chapter 11: Communicating in Primary Care Settings**......... 110

11.1 Addressing Common Acute Illnesses (Colds, Flu, Infections) . 110

11.2 Managing Chronic Conditions (Diabetes, Hypertension, Asthma) ............................................................112

11.3 Providing Preventative Care Advice (Vaccinations, Screenings)
.................................................................... 114

11.4 Discussing Mental Health Concerns ...........................115

Book **6**

## Advanced Healthcare Communication in Spanish

**Chapter 12: Communicating in Emergency Medicine** .........119

12.1 Rapid Assessment and Triage: Asking Crucial Questions Quickly
.................................................................... 119

12.2 Giving Urgent Instructions to Patients and Family Members .121

12.3 Describing Emergency Procedures and Treatments ........ 123

12.4 Communicating with Paramedics and Other Emergency Personnel. . . . . . . . . . . . . . . . . . . . . . . . . . . . . . . . . . . . . . . . . . 124

**Chapter 13: Communicating in Specific Specialties** . . . . . . . . . 127

13.1 Obstetrics and Gynecology: Prenatal Care, Labor and Delivery . . . . . . . . . . . . . . . . . . . . . . . . . . . . . . . . . . . . . . . . . . . . . 127

13.2 Pediatrics: Communicating with Parents and Children. . . . . . 129

13.3 Cardiology: Discussing Heart Conditions and Procedures. . . .131

13.4 Gastroenterology: Explaining Digestive Issues and Treatments . . . . . . . . . . . . . . . . . . . . . . . . . . . . . . . . . . . . . . . . . . . . 134

**Chapter 14: Providing Health Education Materials in Spanish** 142

14.1 Understanding Cultural Considerations in Health Education 142

14.2 Adapting English Materials into Clear and Culturally Sensitive Spanish. . . . . . . . . . . . . . . . . . . . . . . . . . . . . . . . . . . . . . 144

14.3 Explaining Complex Medical Information in Lay Terms. . . . . . 146

14.4 Utilizing Other Educational Resources . . . . . . . . . . . . . . . . . . . 149

**Chapter 15: Conducting Patient Counseling and Motivational Interviewing** . . . . . . . . . . . . . . . . . . . . . . . . . . . . . . . . . . . . . . . . . 151

15.1 Building Trust and Empathy in Counseling Sessions. . . . . . . . .151

15.2 Addressing Patient Fears and Misconceptions . . . . . . . . . . . . . 153

15.3 Using Motivational Interviewing Techniques in Spanish. . . . . 155

15.4 Supporting Patient Adherence to Treatment Plans. . . . . . . . . 156

**Chapter 16: Explaining the Healthcare System to Spanish-Speaking Patients** . . . . . . . . . . . . . . . . . . . . . . . . . . . . . . . . . . . . 159

16.1 Explaining Different Types of Healthcare Providers and Settings . . . . . . . . . . . . . . . . . . . . . . . . . . . . . . . . . . . . . . . . . . . . . . . 159

16.2 Explaining Insurance and Payment Processes . . . . . . . . . . . . .160

16.3 Guiding Patients Through Referrals and Appointments. . . . . 162

Book
**7**

## The Healthcare Professional's Spanish Reference

**Chapter 17: Understanding Common Cultural Beliefs and Practices Related to Health** . . . . . . . . . . . . . . . . . . . . . . . . . . . . . 165

17.1 Family-Centered Decision-Making . . . . . . . . . . . . . . . . . . . . . . . 165

17.2 Recognizing Potential Communication Barriers and How to Overcome Them. . . . . . . . . . . . . . . . . . . . . . . . . . . . . . . . . . . . . . . . . . 167

17.3 Showing Respect for Patient Customs and Traditions . . . . . . .168

17.4 Avoiding Stereotypes and Making Culturally Sensitive Inquiries . . . . . . . . . . . . . . . . . . . . . . . . . . . . . . . . . . . . . . . . . . . . . . . . 170

**Chapter 18: Common Medical Abbreviations and Acronyms in Spanish**. . . . . . . . . . . . . . . . . . . . . . . . . . . . . . . . . . . . . . . . . . . . . . . . 172

**Chapter 19: Trusted Spanish-Language Resources for Healthcare Professionals**. . . . . . . . . . . . . . . . . . . . . . . . . . . . . . . . . . 176

**Chapter 20: Tips for Continued Learning and Language Development** . . . . . . . . . . . . . . . . . . . . . . . . . . . . . . . . . . . . . . . . . 179

## Book 8

## Short Stories in Spanish for Healthcare Professionals

Historia 1: "No es 'nervios', es el corazón" . . . . . . . . . . . . . . . . . . . 183

Historia 2: La receta de la abuela. . . . . . . . . . . . . . . . . . . . . . . . . . . 186

Historia 3: "Solo un susto" . . . . . . . . . . . . . . . . . . . . . . . . . . . . . . . . 189

Historia 4: "¿Me entiende, m'ija?": Construyendo confianza con una paciente mayor y su familia. . . . . . . . . . . . . . . . . . . . . . . . . . 192

Historia 5: El silencio de Carlos . . . . . . . . . . . . . . . . . . . . . . . . . . . 195

Historia 6: "Tengo la presión alta... creo" . . . . . . . . . . . . . . . . . . . 198

Historia 7: "Mi bebé no quiere comer". . . . . . . . . . . . . . . . . . . . . . 201

Historia 8: "Es que trabajo en el campo" . . . . . . . . . . . . . . . . . . . 204

Historia 9: La dieta del "arrocito y pollo" . . . . . . . . . . . . . . . . . . . .207

Historia 10: "No quiero que me pinchen más" . . . . . . . . . . . . . . . . 210

Historia 11: "¿Y eso lo cubre el seguro?" . . . . . . . . . . . . . . . . . . . . 213

Historia 12: "Dice que le duele la panza" . . . . . . . . . . . . . . . . . . . 216

Historia 13: "El papelito lo dice todo" . . . . . . . . . . . . . . . . . . . . . . 219

Historia 14: "Vengo por un chequeo general" . . . . . . . . . . . . . . . .222

Historia 15: "Que Dios la bendiga, doctora". . . . . . . . . . . . . . . . . .225

Appendix A: **Glossary of Common Medical Terms (English – Spanish)**. . . .228

Appendix B: **Common Spanish Phrases for Patient Interactions** . . . . . . . .237

Appendix C: **Bibliography** . . . . . . . . . . . . . . . . . . . . . . . . . . . . . . . .239

**Appendix D: Books by This Author**. . . . . . . . . . . . . . . . . . . . . . . . 240

# $999+ Worth of Extra Resources — At No Extra Cost

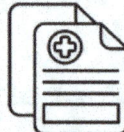

**30+ Patient Communication Sheets (Bilingual)**

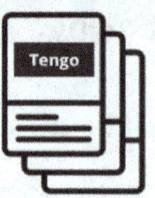

**100 Essential Spanish Verbs – Printable Flashcards**

**2,580 Printable Spanish Flashcards (All Key Topics Covered)**

**40+ Spanish Listening Practice Videos**

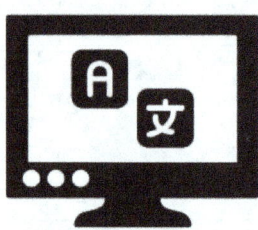

**Spanish Learning Software with 10,000+ Words and Audio Pronunciation**

**Ready to get started? Scan the QR code**

**or visit**
**https://acquirealot.com/getbonus**

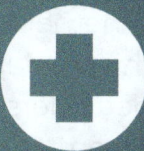

# INTRODUCTION

***Essential Medical Spanish for Healthcare Professionals*** was created to meet a critical and growing need in the healthcare field: effective communication with Spanish-speaking patients. As the population of Spanish speakers continues to expand across many countries, including the United States, healthcare professionals are increasingly called upon to provide care in linguistically and culturally sensitive ways. This book aims to equip providers with the essential language skills, cultural awareness, and clinical communication tools necessary to deliver high-quality care to Spanish-speaking populations.

Caring for patients requires more than language. It's about building trust, understanding their stories, and making complex health issues easier to grasp. A language barrier can often result in misunderstandings, reduced patient satisfaction, and compromised care. ***Essential Medical Spanish for Healthcare Professionals*** is designed to bridge this gap by providing comprehensive, practical, and medically relevant instruction.

This book is the result of combining eight individual volumes into one complete and cohesive resource, each originally designed to address specific areas of Medical Spanish learning. By bringing them together, this edition offers a structured, all-in-one program that supports long-term mastery of both language and clinical communication. It is ideal for self-paced learning, classroom use, or as a professional reference in practice.

The material is laid out in clear, progressive chapters, moving from basic grammar to real conversations you'll have with patients. Each chapter integrates:

- ⊙ Realistic medical dialogues reflecting actual patient-provider interactions.
- ⊙ Targeted grammar explanations focusing on structures commonly used in medical settings.
- ⊙ Pronunciation tips to improve clarity and confidence.
- ⊙ Core vocabulary and essential medical terminology.
- ⊙ Visual aids to support examination procedures and patient education.
- ⊙ Cultural competence considerations to enhance patient rapport and understanding.

Whether you are a physician, nurse, medical student, therapist, or allied health professional, this resource offers a structured approach to mastering Medical Spanish. It is suitable for beginners starting their journey, as well as for experienced providers seeking to refine their communication skills.

Ultimately, **Essential Medical Spanish for Healthcare Professionals** is not just about language acquisition; it is about improving patient outcomes, building stronger provider-patient relationships, and delivering compassionate, effective care. As you work through these chapters, you will develop the confidence to navigate clinical encounters in Spanish with professionalism, accuracy, and empathy.

## A Progressive 15-Minute Daily Plan to Master This Book

The "8 Books in 1" structure of this book is designed for a logical, progressive learning journey. The following 15-minute daily method will allow you to master the material step-by-step, ensuring you build a solid foundation before moving on to more complex clinical conversations.

**The Daily 15-Minute Framework (Your Study Routine):**

- Minutes 1-3: Active Review (Warm-up).
- Before starting a new section, quickly review what you learned the previous day. This reinforces memory and prepares you for the new material.
- Minutes 4-10: New Content (Focus).
- Concentrate on just ONE small section of the chapter you are currently on. The goal is to fully understand a single concept at a time.
- Minutes 11-15: Immediate Practice (Retention).

Apply what you just learned. Say the phrases out loud, cover the Spanish column and test yourself, or complete a related exercise from the book. This active use is crucial for retention.

## How to Progress Through the Book, Chapter by Chapter:

Instead of jumping between books, you will work through the content in the order it is presented. Here's how to apply the 15-minute method:

**1** **Start with the Foundations (Book 1)**

Do not rush through the first book. These are the building blocks for everything that follows. Spend several days or even a full week on Chapter 1.

- **First few days:** Dedicate your 15-minute sessions to "Pronunciation Essentials" (1.3). Practice the pure Spanish vowel sounds and the key consonant differences until they feel natural.
- **Next days:** Move to "Key Linguistic Differences" (1.2). Spend one session on gendered nouns and agreement, and another on formal vs. informal address ("usted" vs. "tú").

- **End the week:** Focus on the "Basic Medical Vocabulary" (1.4) and "Common Grammatical Structures" (1.5). Learn the terms for body parts and practice using verbs like
- *tener, estar,* and *doler.*

### 2  Advance to Clinical Encounters (Book 2)

Once you feel comfortable with the basics, move to the next chapter. For example, when you start Chapter 2: Essential Phrases for Initial Patient Encounters, break it down:

- **Day 1:** Master "Greetings and Introductions" (2.1). Practice the formal phrases aloud.
- **Day 2:** Focus on "Asking for Patient Identification" (2.2). Learn the questions for name, date of birth, and contact information.
- **Day 3:** Work through the "Practical Exercise: Basic Questions in Spanish" (2.6) to test your understanding of the chapter's content.

### 3  Continue the Pattern Systematically

Apply this same method to every chapter. When you reach

**Book 3: Performing the Physical Exam**, spend a 15-minute session learning how to describe the steps (4.1) and the next session practicing how to give instructions for patient positioning (4.2). This ensures you master each skill before adding a new one.

### 4  Use the Stories for Contextual Review (Book 8)

Book 8: Short Stories in Spanish is a powerful tool to consolidate your learning. After completing a book (e.g., after finishing Book 2 on patient history), read a few of the stories. You will see the vocabulary, grammar, and communication strategies you just learned being used in realistic scenarios. For example:

- After learning about pain assessment in Chapter 3, read
- **Historia 12: "Dice que le duele la panza"** to see how a doctor differentiates abdominal pain in a child.
- After studying medication instructions in Book 5, read
- **Historia 6: "Tengo la presión alta... creo"** to understand the challenges of patient adherence and the role of a pharmacist.

By following this progressive method, you will build your Medical Spanish skills on a solid and ever-growing foundation. Each 15-minute session becomes a confident step forward, moving you from basic grammar to complex, empathetic patient communication.

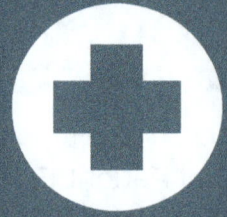

BOOK 1

# FOUNDATIONS OF MEDICAL SPANISH FOR HEALTHCARE PROFESSIONALS

## MASTER ESSENTIAL VOCABULARY AND GRAMMAR FOR CLEAR PATIENT COMMUNICATION

ACQUIRE A LOT

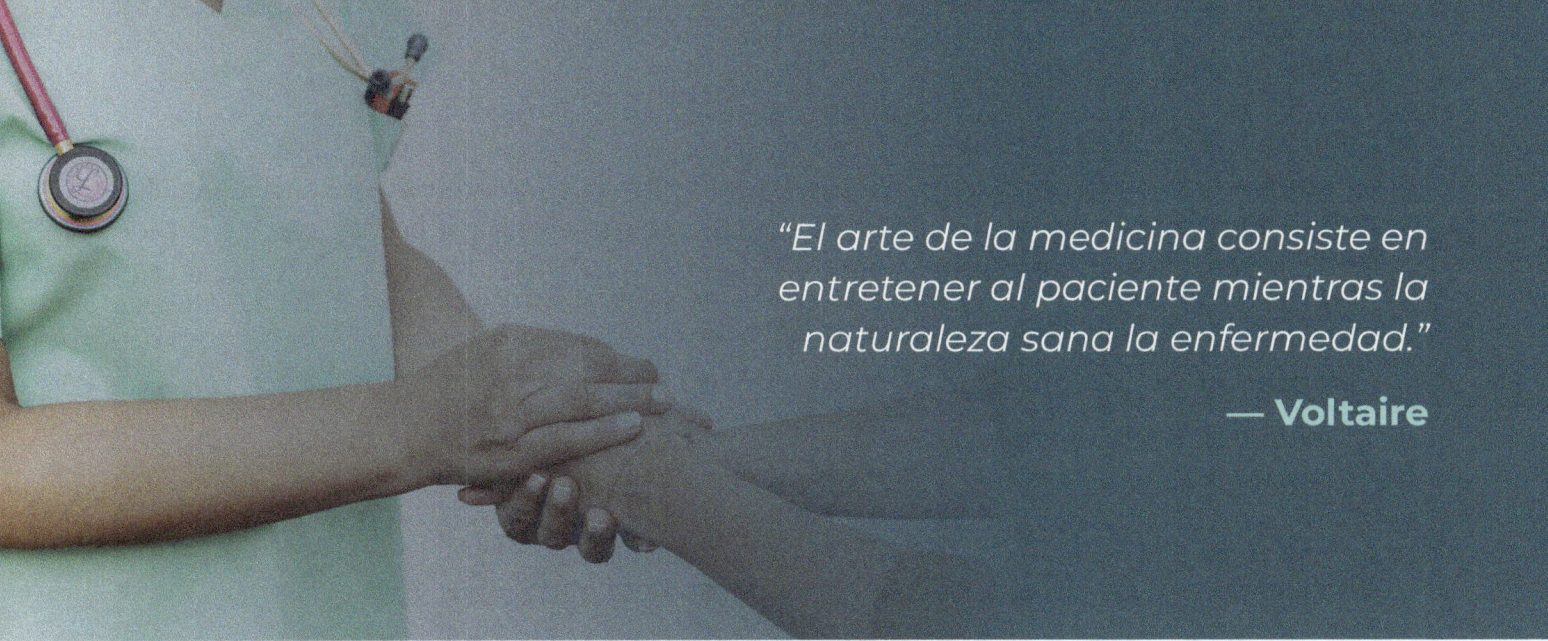

*"El arte de la medicina consiste en entretener al paciente mientras la naturaleza sana la enfermedad."*

**— Voltaire**

CHAPTER 1:

# MEDICAL SPANISH FOR HEALTHCARE PROFESSIONALS

## 1.1 Why Medical Spanish? Meeting the Needs of Spanish-Speaking Patients

In today's diverse healthcare landscape, the ability to communicate across languages is no longer a luxury, it is a necessity. Among the various linguistic groups in the United States and the Americas, Spanish speakers represent one of the largest and fastest-growing populations. This demographic shift presents both an urgent challenge and a unique opportunity for healthcare professionals: the imperative to bridge language gaps through Medical Spanish.

**1  The Demographic Imperative:**

According to U.S. Census data, over 41 million people in the United States speak Spanish at home, and an estimated 25 million are limited English proficient (LEP). Spanish is the most spoken non-English language in the country, and its use is increasing rapidly across all regions, from urban hospitals to rural clinics. As this population continues to expand, the demand for Spanish-language services in healthcare has become not only a matter of efficiency, but of equity, safety, and quality care.

Healthcare providers—whether physicians, nurses, allied health professionals, or administrative staff—are more likely than ever to encounter Spanish-speaking patients in clinical settings. Without adequate language tools, even the most well-intentioned providers may inadvertently contribute to disparities in care.

## 2　The Consequences of Language Barriers:

Language barriers are among the most significant obstacles to effective healthcare delivery. When providers and patients cannot understand each other, the consequences are profound and far-reaching. Miscommunication can lead to:

- Misdiagnoses or incomplete assessments
- Inadequate or misunderstood treatment plans
- Poor medication adherence
- Decreased patient satisfaction
- Higher rates of emergency visits and hospital readmissions
- Legal and ethical vulnerabilities for providers and institutions

## 3　Medical Spanish: A Practical Solution

Importantly, learning Medical Spanish is not about achieving full fluency. Rather, it focuses on building a foundational set of communication tools that enable providers to engage in clear, compassionate, and clinically relevant dialogue. Medical Spanish empowers providers to:

- Ask essential questions during history-taking and triage.
- Explain procedures, diagnoses, medications, and consent forms, avoiding overly technical language when appropriate.
- Provide culturally and spiritually sensitive comfort, reassurance, and support.
- Provide clear discharge instructions and follow-up care plans.
- Recognize and respond to verbal and non-verbal cues specific to Hispanic cultural norms. Here are some common examples:

  - A Hispanic patient — especially a shy one — may avoid eye contact with you and respond repeatedly with "*sí, doctor* or *sí, señor(a)*" even though their body language suggests confusion or discomfort.
  - A Hispanic family member may frequently interrupt to speak on behalf of the patient, even when the patient is capable of answering. This is an expression of protection, not a sign of disrespect.
  - In some Hispanic cultures, people may speak in a loud tone that sometimes could be perceived as shouting even when they are not upset. This is often a normal part of their communication style and not a sign of aggression.

By learning even basic Spanish tailored to healthcare interactions, professionals can dramatically improve their patients' experience and clinical outcomes.

## 4　Enhancing Patient Trust and Reducing Health Disparities

When a provider attempts to speak a patient's language even imperfectly it signals respect, empathy, and a willingness to connect. This simple gesture can build trust, increase compliance with treatment, and foster more open communication. Patients are more likely to share sensitive information, ask questions, and participate in shared decision-making when they feel seen, heard, and respected.

Furthermore, reducing dependence on interpreters for routine interactions can streamline workflows and preserve interpreter services for more complex or legally required situations. It also allows for more immediate responses in challenging environments like emergency rooms or urgent care.

### 5  Promoting Health Equity:

Language access is a core part of health equity. Without it, Spanish-speaking patients are at a structural disadvantage in a system that often defaults to English. Medical Spanish education represents a meaningful step toward correcting this imbalance.

Institutions that support bilingual or multilingual training contribute to a more inclusive, patient-centered model of care. Individual providers who invest in language learning not only elevate their clinical competence but also help close the gap in healthcare disparities affecting Latino and Spanish-speaking communities.

### 6  A Call to Action:

Learning Medical Spanish is an investment in your professional development—and more importantly, in your patients. This book will guide you through the foundational skills needed to begin or enhance your ability to communicate in Spanish. With each phrase learned and each encounter improved, you become part of a broader movement toward safer, more effective, and providing culturally sensitive care.

## 1.2 Key Linguistic Differences Between English and Medical Spanish

To communicate effectively in a medical setting, healthcare professionals must do more than translate words they must understand how Spanish functions as a language, especially within clinical contexts. Medical Spanish is not merely a direct conversion of English medical terminology. It involves distinct structural, grammatical, and cultural features that, when properly understood, significantly improve clarity, reduce miscommunication, and foster patient trust.

While conversational Spanish may be sufficient for informal interactions, medical Spanish demands a higher level of precision and formality. This section outlines the most important linguistic differences between English and Spanish that impact healthcare communication, offering healthcare professionals a foundational understanding of how to navigate patient encounters more confidently and accurately.

### 1  Word Order: Reversed Placement of Descriptive Words

One of the most noticeable differences between English and Spanish is the order in which adjectives and nouns appear. In English, adjectives typically precede the nouns they describe ("abdominal pain"), whereas in Spanish, the order is reversed ("*dolor abdominal*").

Examples:

- *Dolor abdominal* — abdominal pain.
- *Presión* alta — high blood pressure.
- *Fiebre leve* — mild fever.

## 2 Gendered Nouns and Agreement

Spanish nouns are gendered, meaning they are classified as either masculine or feminine.

This classification affects not only the articles ("el" for masculine, "la" for feminine) but also the adjectives and past participles associated with them. English does not have grammatical gender, which often leads to confusion for new Spanish learners.

Examples:

- El brazo roto. — The broken arm.
- La pierna hinchada. — the swollen leg.
- La infección grave. — the serious infection.
- El paciente enfermo. — The sick (male) patient.
- La paciente embarazada. — The pregnant patient
- El médico. — The male doctor.
- La médica. — The female doctor.
- El niño enfermo — The sick boy.
- La niña enferma — The sick girl.

## 3 Formal Register: Using "Usted" in Medical Settings

A key element of professionalism in Spanish-language communication is the use of the formal second-person pronoun "*usted*" instead of the informal "tú". The choice of pronouns impacts verb conjugation and tone. In medical environments, particularly when addressing adult patients, elders, or in formal settings such as hospitals and clinics, "*usted*" is the expected form. It communicates respect and maintains professional boundaries.

Common examples:

- *¿Cómo se siente usted hoy?* — *How are you feeling today?*
- *¿Tiene usted alguna alergia?* — *Do you have any allergies?*
- *Le voy a tomar la presión arterial.* — *I'm going to take your blood pressure.*

It can also be correct to omit the formal "*usted*" in a formal sentence. For example:

- *¿Cómo se siente hoy?* — *How are you feeling today?*
- *¿Tiene alguna alergia?* — *Do you have any allergies?*

**Cultural Note:** The Use of Don and Doña in Latin America[2]

In many Latin American cultures, addressing someone as "Don" or "Doña" followed by their first name — for example, "Don José" or "Doña María" — communicates not only respect, but also warmth and familiarity, especially toward older adults. These honorifics have roots in colonial social hierarchies (dominus/domina in Latin), but today their meaning is more symbolic, often tied to age, social standing, or a person's role within the community.

In rural areas or among older generations, Don and Doña are commonly used to acknowledge someone's status, experience, or seniority. Sometimes, they may even serve as informal titles of leadership or reference, similar to calling someone "boss" or "elder."

However, their use is not universal. In more urban or professional settings — such as hospitals or clinics — Don and Doña may sound outdated or overly informal, particularly when addressing younger adults. In these contexts, it's often more appropriate to use "señor" or "señora" followed by the last name.

A helpful strategy to choose the most appropriate form of address is to listen carefully to how the patient is referred to by family members or close companions. For example, if a son-in-law calls her Doña, that is a clear cultural cue that this form of address is both appropriate and expected. The same applies when someone is referred to as Don — it usually signals a respectful, socially accepted way of addressing the person.

 **4    False Cognates:** Tricky Look-Alikes

False cognates, or "false friends," are words that look similar in English and Spanish but have different meanings. In healthcare, relying on visual similarity without understanding true meaning can result in serious miscommunication.

**Common False Cognates in Medical Settings:**

False cognates are words that look or sound similar in two languages —in this case, English and Spanish — but have different meanings. In medical contexts, these misleading similarities can cause confusion between healthcare providers and patients, particularly when Spanish-speaking patients assume that a familiar-sounding English word means the same as its Spanish counterpart. Such misunderstandings can lead to inaccurate documentation, misinterpretation of symptoms or instructions, and ultimately impact patient safety, trust, and quality of care. For this reason, recognizing and clarifying false cognates is essential in cross-cultural communication within healthcare settings.

Below you'll find a table showing the most common cognates in English and Spanish used in the healthcare setting.

# False Cognates in Medicine: Commonly Confused Terms

| Español / Spanish | Se confunde con... / Mistaken for... | En realidad significa... / Actually means... | Traducción real de la palabra inglesa / Actual meaning of mistaken English word |
|---|---|---|---|
| Asistir | to assist | to attend (asistir a clase — to attend class) | to assist — ayudar |
| Actualmente | actually | currently | actually — en realidad |
| Embarazada (*) | embarrassed | pregnant | embarrassed — avergonzado/a |
| Constipado (*) | constipated | having a cold / nasal congestion | constipated — estreñido |
| Sensible | sensible | sensitive | sensible — sensato / prudente |
| Molestar (*) | to molest | to bother / to annoy | to molest — abusar sexualmente |
| Intoxicado | intoxicated | food or chemical poisoning | intoxicated — ebrio / bajo efectos del alcohol o drogas ilícitas |
| Ropa | rope | clothes | rope — cuerda |
| Éxito | exit | success | exit — salida |
| Sano | sane | healthy | sane — mentalmente estable |
| Firma | firm | signature | firm — empresa |
| Discutir | to discuss | to argue (confrontar o debatir acaloradamente) | to discuss — conversar / analizar |
| Realizar | to realize | to carry out / to perform | to realize — darse cuenta |
| Recordar | to record | to remember | to record — grabar |

**(*) Cultural Notes**: Perhaps the three most frequent false cognates that cause confusion for English speakers learning medical Spanish are *"embarazada,"* *"constipado,"* and *"molestar."* While they may resemble familiar English words, their actual meanings are quite different and in clinical settings, these misunderstandings can lead to awkward or even serious consequences.

"*Embarazada*" means pregnant, not embarrassed. This is a classic error in class and clinical practice. The correct way to say embarrassed is "*avergonzado/a.*"

"*Constipado*" refers to having a cold or nasal congestion, not being constipated. The proper term for constipated is "*estreñido/a.*"

"*Molestar*" is another tricky one. In Spanish, it simply means to bother or to annoy — as in "*¿Le molesta la luz?*" (Does the light bother you?). However, in English, "to molest" carries a very serious and inappropriate meaning related to sexual abuse. It's important to be aware of this difference to avoid misunderstandings and maintain patient trust.

## 5   Medical Terminology: Latin Roots and Clarity

Many English and Spanish medical terms share Latin roots, resulting in terminology that is often similar in both languages. This linguistic connection can be a valuable aid for healthcare professionals working in bilingual environments, as recognizing these shared roots can support clearer communication and facilitate learning. While caution is needed to avoid false cognates, true cognates—words that share both form and meaning—are particularly helpful in understanding and explaining medical concepts.

The following table lists common cognates (true cognates) in English and Spanish used in medical contexts.

### True Cognates in Medicine

| Español / Spanish | Inglés / English |
| --- | --- |
| Diabetes | Diabetes |
| Anemia | Anemia |
| Fractura | Fracture |
| Hipertensión arterial | High blood pressure / Hypertension |
| Síndrome del túnel carpiano | Carpal tunnel syndrome |
| Infección del tracto urinario | Urinary tract infection |
| Bronquitis | Bronchitis |
| Hepatitis | Hepatitis |
| Gastritis | Gastritis |
| Migraña | Migraine |
| Alergia | Allergy |
| Cirrosis | Cirrhosis |

### 6  Why These Differences Matter in Clinical Practice

These linguistic differences are not mere academic curiosities they have real implications for the quality of patient care. A provider who uses accurate word order, honors grammatical gender, speaks in an appropriately formal register, and avoids common false cognates is more likely to earn their patient's trust and deliver care that is both safe and effective.

Moreover, understanding the structure and rhythm of Spanish allows healthcare professionals to listen more effectively. Recognizing patterns such as adjective placement or verb conjugation helps providers process what the patient is saying and respond in ways that confirm understanding and compassion.

## 1.3 Pronunciation Essentials for Clear Communication

Clear pronunciation is a cornerstone of effective communication in any language, and this is particularly true in healthcare, where accuracy and clarity can significantly affect patient outcomes.

One of the advantages of Spanish, compared to English, is its phonetic consistency words are typically pronounced just as they are spelled. However, for English-speaking healthcare providers, understanding the key differences and rules of Spanish pronunciation is critical to achieving mutual understanding with patients and avoiding potentially serious misunderstandings.

Spanish pronunciation, while more consistent than English, requires specific attention to vowels, consonants, syllable stress, and the avoidance of Anglicized pronunciations, especially when using medical terminology. Developing a clear and confident Spanish pronunciation not only increases a provider's confidence but also promotes trust and comfort in Spanish-speaking patients.

### 1  Vowel Clarity: Five Pure Sounds

Spanish has five vowels: a, e, i, o, and u. Each vowel has a single, pure sound, unlike English vowels, which often vary depending on context and are frequently diphthongized.

Examples:

- a — ah (as in "father") — *garganta* (throat)
- e — eh (as in "bed") — *enfermero* (nurse)
- i — ee (as in "machine") — *infección* (infection)
- o — oh (as in "hope") — *dolor* (pain)
- u — oo (as in "flute") — *tumor* (tumor)

These vowel sounds never change, regardless of their position in a word. Accurate vowel pronunciation ensures intelligibility and avoids confusion. Mispronouncing even a single vowel can render a term unrecognizable to native speakers.

## 2 Consonant Differences: Key Articulations to Learn

While many Spanish consonants are like their English counterparts, several require special attention:

- ⊙ r / rr: The single "r" is tapped lightly (as in "*pero*"), while the double "rr" is trilled (as in "*perro*"). The single "r" is also trilled when it is at the beginning of a word—for example, "*rojo*" red). Mispronouncing this can change meanings entirely.

- ⊙ g: Pronounced as a soft "h" sound before "e" or "i" (as in *gente*), but like the English "g" in "go" before other vowels.

- ⊙ j: Pronounced like a strong English "h," as in *jarabe* (syrup).

- ⊙ ñ: A nasal sound similar to "ny" in "canyon," used in words like *niño* (child).

- ⊙ h: Always silent in Spanish, even in medical terms like *hospital* (ohs-pee-TAHL).

Attention to these details improves clarity and minimizes patient confusion, especially when delivering sensitive or critical health information.

## 3 Syllable Stress:

Knowing Where the Emphasis Falls Proper syllable stress is vital to ensure that words are understood correctly. In Spanish, there are general rules for stress:

- ⊙ If a word ends in a vowel, "n," or "s," stress naturally falls on the second-to-last (penultimate) syllable.

- ⊙ If a word ends in any other consonant, stress falls on the last syllable.

- ⊙ If stress is irregular, it will be indicated by an accent mark (e.g., *fácil*, *infección*, *pólipo*).

Incorrect stress can change a word's meaning or make it difficult for the listener to understand. For instance, *pico* (beak/peak) vs. *picó* (he/she stung), or *medico* (I medicate) vs. *médico* (doctor).

## 4 Avoiding Common Mispronunciations: Don't Anglicize

It's very common for English-speaking learners to pronounce Spanish words using English sounds—especially when the words look familiar, like many medical terms do. This happens because English and Spanish share many roots, and it's easy to assume they're pronounced the same way. The good news is that with just a bit of practice, adjusting pronunciation can make a big difference. Saying words the way patients expect to hear them not only improves understanding, but also shows kindness, cultural respect, and a real commitment to connecting. In healthcare, these small efforts go a long way in making patients feel seen, heard, and safe.

The following is a list of commonly used medical terms with their correct pronunciation, along with helpful tips

## Pronunciation Guide for Common Medical Term

| Term | Mispronunciation (Anglicized) | Correct Pronunciation | Notes |
|---|---|---|---|
| Diabetes | Dee-ah-betis | Dya-be-tehs | Stress on the third syllable in Spanish. |
| Hipertensión | Hy-per-ten-see-own | Ee-per-ten-syon | Avoid English diphthongs and the "H" sound. |
| Infección urinaria | In-fek-shun del tracto yoo-ree-nay-ree-o | Een-fek-syon del trak-to u-ree-na-rio | Keep Spanish vowel sounds short and pure. |
| Gastritis | Gas-try-tis | Gas-tree-tees | Spanish stress on penultimate syllable. |
| Sinusitis | Sigh-nus-itis | See-noo-see-tees | Use consistent vowel sounds. |
| Nefrología | Knee-fro-lo-gee | Neh-fro-lo-hee-a | Avoid anglicizing the "-gía" ending. |
| Anemia | An-ee-mee-uh | Ah-ne-mee-a | Use clear Spanish vowel sounds. |
| Obesidad | Oh-bee-sitty | Oh-bee-see-dad | Don't confuse "-dad" with the English "-ty". |
| Embarazada | Em-buh-rah-zay-duh | Em-ba-ra-sa-da | Do not confuse it with "embarazoso", which means "embarrassing." |
| Colon | Kow-lon or Co-lin | Ko-lon | Use a short, clear "o" in both syllables; not pronounced like "colonel." |
| Cirugía | Sir-yu-gee-uh | See-roo-hee-a | Soft "gía" ending; avoid "gee-uh" sound. |
| Medicación | Med-ee-kay-shun | Me-dee-ka-syon | Keep Spanish syllable pattern and avoid the "-shun" English ending. |

Spanish speakers, in general, tend to be empathetic and receptive when someone makes the effort to communicate in Spanish, even if they make mistakes or have a strong accent. This attitude reflects deeply rooted cultural values such as warmth, politeness, and appreciation for human connection. Especially in sensitive settings like healthcare, Spanish-speaking patients often greatly value when a healthcare professional tries to speak their language, as it is seen as a gesture of respect, closeness, and genuine care — which significantly strengthens the patient-provider relationship, builds trust, and improves collaboration in treatment. It also helps reduce patient anxiety and contributes to a more human and compassionate experience.

### 5 Building Pronunciation Skills Through Active Practice

Developing clear pronunciation is a skill built through repeated exposure and deliberate practice.

Techniques include:

- Listening to native Spanish speakers through medical videos, podcasts, or language learning apps
- Practicing aloud with a focus on vowels, stress, and rhythm
- Using repetition drills with medical vocabulary and phrases
- Engaging in role-play or guided dialogues with feedback from fluent speakers

## 1.4 Basic Medical Vocabulary: Core Terms and Concepts

Medical Spanish begins with a foundation of essential vocabulary that allows healthcare professionals to participate in basic clinical conversations. Whether asking a patient where it hurts, understanding reported symptoms, or identifying staff roles and locations within a hospital, knowing the correct terms in Spanish is vital for safe and effective care.

While grammar and pronunciation shape how words are used, vocabulary forms the building blocks of communication. In this section, we explore the core categories of medical terminology that appear frequently in patient interactions.

Mastery of these terms improves provider confidence and enables more fluid, respectful, and empathetic exchanges in Spanish-speaking environments.

### 1 Body Parts: Building Anatomical Awareness

Understanding and correctly naming body parts in Spanish allows providers to describe, assess, and localize symptoms or conditions. Anatomical terms are often used in triage, exams, and patient instructions.

Some common body parts:

- *Cabeza* — Head
- *Estómago* — Stomach
- *Pecho* — Chest
- *Pierna* — Leg
- *Brazo* — Arm

- *Espalda* — Back
- *Riñón* — Kidney
- *Abdomen* — Abdomen
- *Corazón* — Heart

- *Cuello* — Neck (external part)
- *Garganta* — Throat (internal part, including pharynx/larynx)

Using precise anatomical terms reduces ambiguity and enhances clarity when patients describe symptoms, point to pain, or ask for explanations. In some contexts, *"cuello"* (neck) and *"garganta"* (throat) can appear to be interchangeable in Spanish, especially in everyday speech. However, medically speaking, they refer to distinct anatomical areas and should be used precisely to avoid confusion.

## 2  Symptoms: Recognizing Common Complaints

Symptom-related vocabulary is critical in early clinical encounters, especially when identifying the chief complaint, understanding the history of present illness, or evaluating treatment response. It helps providers ask clearer questions, interpret answers accurately, and build trust through effective communication.

Examples of useful symptoms:

- *Dolor* — Pain
- *Náusea* — Nausea
- *Fiebre* — Fever
- *Tos* — Cough
- *Mareo* — Dizziness or lightheadedness
- *Vómito* — Vomiting
- *Dificultad para respirar* — Difficulty breathing
- *Congestión nasal* — Nasal congestion / Stuffy nose
- *Diarrea* — Diarrhea
- *Dolor muscular* — Myalgia
- *Pérdida del conocimiento* — Loss of consciousness

These terms support the identification of potential red flags and help providers prioritize care based on acuity and severity.

## 3  Vital Signs: Monitoring the Basics

Vital signs are universal indicators of a patient's physiological status. Being able to refer to them in Spanish helps providers explain procedures and share findings.

Common vital signs are:

- *Presión arterial* — Blood pressure
- *Temperatura corporal* — Body temperature
- *Frecuencia cardíaca* — Heart rate
- *Frecuencia respiratoria* — Respiratory rate
- *Saturación de oxígeno* — Oxygen saturation
- *Nivel del dolor* — Pain level

These words are especially useful in initial assessments, patient education, and follow-up conversations about treatment responses.

## 4  Medical Personnel and Settings: Navigating the Environment

Healthcare involves a wide network of people and locations. Knowing how to identify key personnel and clinical areas in Spanish aids orientation and coordination, especially in hospitals or multi-provider clinics.

In Spanish, you would say:

- *Médico/médica* — doctor/physician
- *Especialista* — specialist
- *Enfermero/enfermera* — nurse
- *Intérprete* — interpreter
- *Farmacia* — pharmacy
- *Clínica* — clinic

*Essential Medical Spanish for Healthcare Professionals*

- *Urgencias* — emergency room
- *Sala de espera* — waiting room
- *Sala de cirugía* — surgery room.

These terms allow for smoother transitions between departments and support patients in understanding their care pathway.

### 5 Basic Verbs: Essential Actions in Clinical Contexts

Verbs are essential for forming questions, giving instructions, and describing symptoms or actions. A small set of high-frequency verbs carries a wide range of clinical utility.

These are some examples of how to use basic verbs

- *Tener* — to have (used to: explore symptoms or medical conditions: *"Tengo fiebre."* – I have a fever. "
- *¿Le han diagnosticado alguna enfermedad?"* – Have you been diagnosed with any illnesses?)
- *Sentir(se)* — to feel (e.g., *"¿Cómo se siente?"* – How do you feel? It can refer to both physical and emotional state).
- *Doler* — to hurt (e.g., *"¿Le duele?"* – Does it hurt?)
- *Tomar* — to take (used for medication or vital signs)
- *Necesitar* — to need (e.g., *"¿Necesita ayuda?"* – Do you need help?)
- *Padecer / sufrir* — to suffer from (e.g., *"¿Padece alguna enfermedad?"* – Do you suffer from any condition?)

## 1.5 Common Grammatical Structures in Medical Contexts

In clinical environments, the primary objective of Medical Spanish is not grammatical perfection but effective communication. Healthcare professionals must be able to convey information clearly, understand patient concerns, and give instructions confidently. Mastering a select group of essential grammatical patterns allows clinicians to manage a wide range of medical scenarios with greater ease.

### 1 Using the Verb "Tener" (To Have) for Symptoms

In Spanish, many symptoms are expressed using the verb *tener* ("to have") instead of *"ser"* or *"estar"* ("to be"), reflecting both a structural and conceptual difference from English. In English, physical states are commonly described using the verb to be, as in "I am cold" or "I am sick", which convey a temporary condition affecting the subject.

In contrast, Spanish speakers use *tener* to express these same ideas, saying *tengo frío* (literally, "I have cold"), *tengo hambre* ("I have hunger"), or tengo una *enfermedad* ("I have an illness"). This difference highlights how Spanish tends to conceptualize many physical or symptomatic conditions as things a person possesses, rather than as states of being.

Sample questions using "*tener*":

- ⊙ *¿Tiene fiebre?* — Do you have a fever?
- ⊙ *Tengo dolor de garganta.* — I have a sore throat.
- ⊙ *¿Tiene náusea o vómito?* — Do you have nausea or vomiting?

"*Tener*" is used with a wide range of symptom expressions and is foundational to initial patient assessment. However, the verbs "*estar*" or "*ser*" can also be used in certain contexts instead of "*tener*", depending on regional variation or emphasis.

Sample questions using "*estar*" or "*ser*":

- ⊙ *Estoy con frío.* — I am cold.
- ⊙ *Soy hipertenso.* — I have High Blood Pressure.
- ⊙ *Estoy con dolor en la pierna.* — I have pain in my leg.
- ⊙ Soy diabético tipo 2 — I have type 2 diabetes.

### 2  Using the Verb "Estar" (To Be) for Temporary States

The verb "estar" is used to describe temporary or changing conditions. This includes how the patient feels in the moment, their physical state, or location.

Useful phrases:

- ⊙ *Está mareado.* — He/She is dizzy.
- ⊙ *Estoy cansada.* — I am tired. (spoken by a female)
- ⊙ *¿Tiene dolor? / ¿Siente dolor?* — Are you in pain?
- ⊙ *¿Está usted bien?* — Are you okay?
- ⊙ *¿Esto duele?* — Does this hurt? (e.g., when palpating the abdomen)

This verb is especially important in emergency or acute care settings where the patient's current condition is being evaluated.

### 3  Expressing Pain using "*Doler*" and Reflexive Structures

Spanish expresses pain using a structure that may seem unfamiliar to English speakers. The verb "*doler*" (to hurt) functions similarly to "*gustar,*" requiring an indirect object pronoun.

Useful phrases:

- ⊙ *Me duele la cabeza.* — My head hurts. (Literally: The head hurts me.)
- ⊙ *¿Le duele aquí?* — Does it hurt here?
- ⊙ *Nos duelen los pies.* — Our feet hurt.

This structure is a staple of clinical interviews and should be practiced regularly for fluency and comprehension.

**4** **Giving Instructions with Command Forms (Imperatives)**

In clinical settings, clear and respectful instructions are vital. Spanish uses the imperative mood to issue commands, most often in the formal usted form.

Sample expressions:

- *Respire profundo.* — Take a deep breath.
- *Abra la boca.* — Open your mouth.
- *Mueva el cuello.* — Move your neck.
- *Quédese quieto.* — Stay still.

Command forms must be delivered with the correct tone and verb form to avoid sounding abrupt or impolite. In some cases, you may choose to use a more polite or indirect tone. For example:

- *¿Puede mover su brazo?* — Can you move your arm?
- *Por favor, mueva el cuello* — Please move your neck.
- *¿Por favor, puede quedarse quieto? / ¿Puede quedarse quieto, por favor?* — Could you stay still, please?

These softer forms can enhance rapport with patients, especially in sensitive situations or with those who may feel anxious.

**5** **Asking Questions Using Inversion**

Spanish uses subject-verb inversion in many types of questions, especially yes/no questions. Understanding this structure allows providers to ask clear and grammatically accurate questions.

Sample expressions:

- *¿Le duele aquí?* — Does it hurt here?
- *¿Tiene usted alergias? / ¿Sufre de alergias?* — Do you have any allergies?
- *¿Está tomando medicamentos?* — Are you taking any medications?
- These forms are essential for history taking, medication review, and patient monitoring.

**6** **Showing Respect with the Formal "*Usted*" Form**

Spanish distinguishes between formal and informal speech. In healthcare, the formal "usted" form should be used when addressing adult patients, families, and elders to convey professionalism and respect.

Appropriate wording:

- *¿Cómo se siente usted hoy?* — How are you feeling today?
- *¿Desea sentarse?* — Would you like to sit down?
- *¿Puede decirme qué pasó / ¿Puede decirme qué ocurrió?* — Can you tell me what happened?

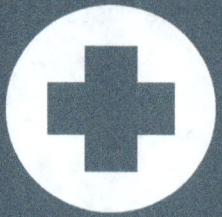

BOOK 2

# CLINICAL
# CONSULTATION
# IN SPANISH

## A HEALTHCARE GUIDE FOR
## INITIAL PATIENT ENCOUNTERS
## AND HISTORY TAKING

ACQUIRE A LOT

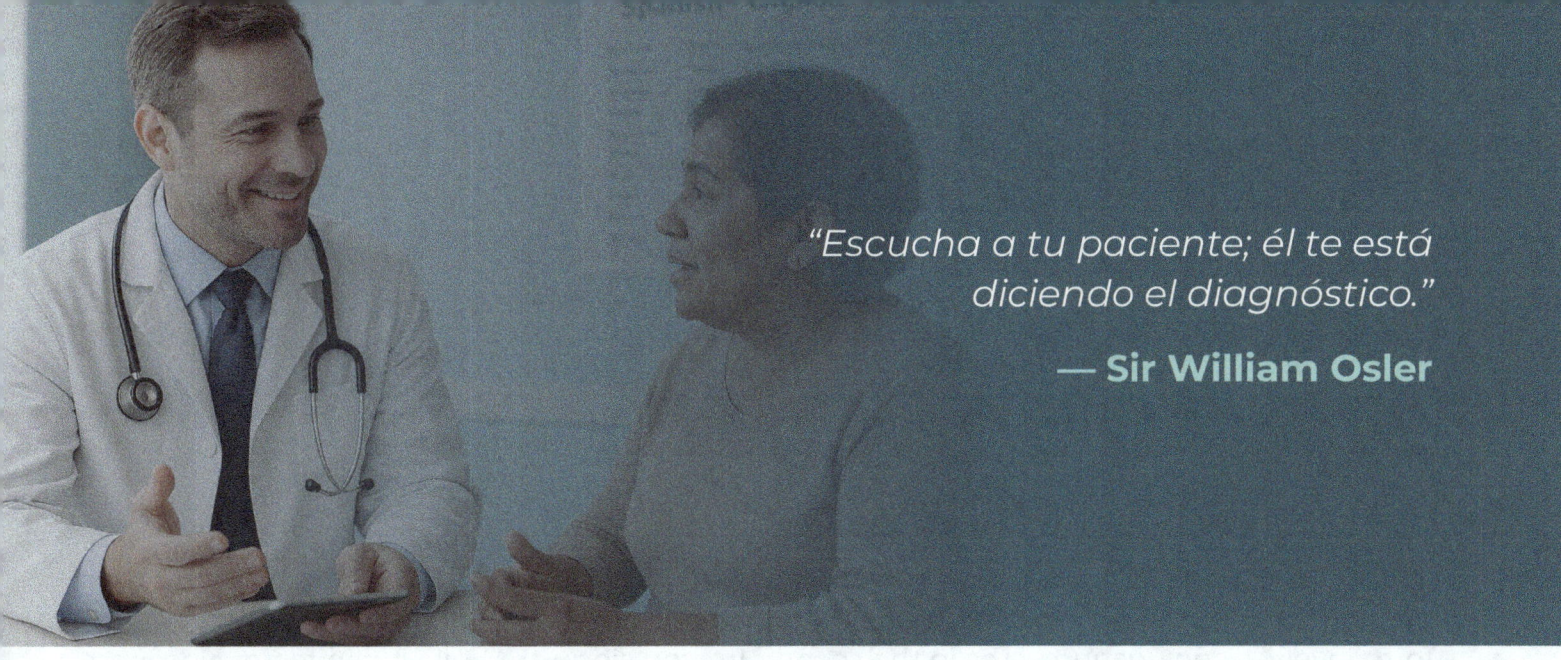

*"Escucha a tu paciente; él te está diciendo el diagnóstico."*

— **Sir William Osler**

CHAPTER 2:

# ESSENTIAL PHRASES FOR INITIAL PATIENT ENCOUNTERS

## 2.1 Greetings and Introductions: Formal and Informal

Good communication starts with a warm, culturally sensitive greeting. The initial moments of a patient-provider interaction set the tone for the entire clinical encounter. Whether assessing a new patient in the emergency room or following up in a primary care setting, how a healthcare professional introduces themselves has a significant impact on trust, comfort, and rapport.

In Spanish-speaking cultures, greetings carry strong social significance and are often more formal than in English-speaking settings. A warm, respectful introduction not only honors cultural expectations but also reflects professionalism and empathy.

In Spanish, speakers distinguish between formal and informal ways of addressing others, depending on the context, the level of familiarity, and the need to show respect. This chapter reviews key structures and phrases for both types of greetings and introduces the important concept of individuals' preferred names.

### 1  Formal Greetings in Clinical Settings

As a rule, healthcare providers should use formal language. This style of speech demonstrates respect, especially when addressing adults, elders, or individuals who are not personally known. In Spanish, formal language involves the use of the pronoun "usted" and its corresponding third-person singular verb forms. It is commonly used in medical settings to maintain professionalism and a respectful distance.

Model phrases:

- *Buenos días, soy el doctor García.* — Good morning, I'm Dr. García.
- *Buenas tardes, soy la enfermera López.* — Good afternoon, I'm Nurse López.
- *Hola, mucho gusto. ¿Cómo está usted?* — Hi, nice to meet you. How are you?
- *Buenos días, ¿cómo se siente hoy?* — Good morning, how are you feeling today?

These phrases establish a respectful tone and are appropriate for all professional healthcare environments, including hospitals, clinics, and home visits.

### 2  Informal Greetings: When Appropriate

Informal language in Spanish is generally used with people you know well—such as long-term patients, children, or individuals who clearly indicate a preference for informal speech. The "tú" form involves conjugating verbs in the second person singular. While it can foster closeness, it should never be assumed without cultural or contextual cues.

Healthcare providers should remain sensitive to the clinical setting, the patient's age, cultural background, and the expected formality of the interaction. When in doubt, it is best to begin formally and adjust based on the patient's comfort and communication style.

Below is a chart with example phrases that illustrate the difference between formal and informal interactions in Spanish.

#### Formal vs. Informal Spanish Phrases

| Español / Spanish | Tipo / Type | Inglés / English |
|---|---|---|
| ¿Cómo estás? | Informal | How are you? |
| ¿Cómo está usted? / ¿Cómo está? | Formal | |
| ¿Tienes dolor? | Informal | Do you have pain? |
| ¿Tiene algún síntoma? | Formal | Do you have any symptoms? |
| Hola, ¿cómo está? / ¿Hola, cómo se encuentra? | Formal | Hi, how are you? |
| Hola, ¿cómo estás? / ¿Hola, cómo te encuentras? | Informal | |
| Me llamo Ana y soy la enfermera que te atenderá. Mucho gusto. | Informal | I'm the nurse who will be taking care of you. My name is Ana. Nice to meet you. |
| Mucho gusto, soy Ana y seré la enfermera que lo atenderá. | Formal | |
| ¿Te sientes mejor hoy? | Informal | Are you feeling better today? |

### 3  Asking for Preferred Names

A respectful introduction includes not only presenting oneself professionally but also inquiring how the patient prefers to be addressed. This small gesture can make patients feel seen, respected, and involved in their care.

Language examples:

- *¿Cómo prefiere que le llame?* — How do you prefer to be addressed?
- *¿Quiere que le llame señora Martínez o María?* — Would you like me to call you Mrs. Martínez or María?

This is especially relevant in diverse cultural and gender identity contexts, where formal titles or legal names may not reflect a patient's preferences.

### 4  Introducing Others and Clarifying Roles

Clarity around roles enhances trust and reduces confusion. Patients often interact with multiple providers during a visit, so brief introductions help clarify who is responsible for what.

Language examples:

- *Ella es la doctora Rivera, especialista en cardiología.* — She is Dr. Rivera, a cardiologist.
- *Este es el técnico que le hará la radiografía.* — *This is the* technician who will take your X-ray.
- *Yo soy su intérprete médico.* — I'm your medical interpreter.

A simple introduction can make a big difference. It helps the patient feel seen, supported, and cared for.

## 2.2 Asking for Patient Identification and Basic Information

Accurate patient identification is a critical first step in any healthcare encounter. Confirming a patient's identity is essential not only for legal and safety reasons but also for building a relationship grounded in trust and respect. In Spanish-speaking settings, healthcare providers must be equipped to ask for identifying details clearly, respectfully, and in a culturally appropriate manner.

Asking for basic details—name, birth date, contact, ID—helps avoid mistakes and keeps care on track This first exchange helps create a professional, clear atmosphere.

### 1  Asking for Full Name

Establishing identity begins with the patient's full legal name. In many Spanish-speaking cultures, individuals may use two surnames (one paternal, one maternal), and this naming convention should be respected in documentation.

Common phrases:

- ⊙ *¿Cuál es su nombre completo?* — What is your full name?
- ⊙ *¿Cómo se escribe su apellido?* — How do you spell your last name?
- ⊙ *¿Tiene otro nombre o apodo que prefiera usar?* — Do you have another name or nickname you prefer to use?

Being attentive to how names are used and pronounced shows cultural sensitivity and helps avoid clerical errors.

## 2 Confirming Date of Birth

The patient's date of birth is often used to confirm identity in healthcare systems. This information must be communicated clearly and double-checked for accuracy, as errors can lead to serious issues in recordkeeping, medication administration, or treatment planning.

For elderly patients in particular, it is important to verify the date of birth against a photo ID or, when necessary, with a family member or caregiver. Age-related conditions such as memory loss, confusion, or hearing impairment may affect a patient's ability to recall or communicate this information accurately. Confirming it through reliable sources helps ensure safety, proper documentation, and respectful care.

How to word it:

- ⊙ *¿Cuál es su fecha de nacimiento?* — What is your date of birth?
- ⊙ *¿En qué año nació?* — What year were you born?
- ⊙ *¿Puede repetir su fecha de nacimiento, por favor?* — Can you repeat your date of birth, please?

Keep in mind that date formats vary across cultures. In the United States, dates are typically written as month-day-year (MM/DD/YYYY), whereas in most Latin American countries, the format is day-month-year (DD/MM/YYYY). Always clarify the order if there is any risk of confusion, especially when recording dates in medical records or scheduling procedures.

## 3 Requesting Photo Identification

When appropriate, verifying the patient's identity using an official document such as a government-issued ID helps confirm patient records and insurance information.

For instance, you would say:

- ⊙ *¿Tiene una identificación con foto?* — Do you have a photo ID?
- ⊙ *¿Puedo ver su tarjeta de seguro médico?* — May I see your health insurance card?
- ⊙ *¿Trajo algún documento de identidad?* — Did you bring any form of identification?

Asking for identification should always be done respectfully, especially if a patient expresses concern about privacy, immigration status, or document availability.

**4** **Collecting Contact Information**

Gathering contact details ensures that providers can follow up regarding test results, appointments, or billing inquiries. Accuracy in this area is essential for continuity of care.

Common phrases used to collect information:

- *¿Cuál es su dirección?* — What is your address?
- *¿Cuál es su correo electrónico?* — What is your email address?
- *¿Cuál es su número de teléfono?* — What is your phone number?
- *¿Tiene otro número de contacto?* — Do you have another contact number?
- *¿Vive usted solo o con familia?* — Do you live alone or with family?

Understanding a patient's living situation can provide useful context for care planning, particularly in cases of chronic illness or home-based care.

## 2.3 Establishing Rapport and Addressing Patient Comfort

Establishing rapport and ensuring patient comfort are critical components of quality care. For Spanish-speaking patients, culturally sensitive communication and genuine expressions of empathy can significantly influence their willingness to participate in their care and follow medical advice. In many healthcare encounters, anxiety, uncertainty, or fear can function as barriers to trust. By creating a welcoming and respectful environment, healthcare professionals not only improve patient satisfaction but also increase the likelihood of positive clinical outcomes.

In Spanish-speaking cultures, warmth and attentive respect go a long way. A provider's ability to demonstrate compassion through language—verbal and nonverbal—strengthens the therapeutic alliance.

**1** **Asking About Comfort**

Checking in with the patient's physical and emotional comfort is a simple but powerful way to begin any interaction. This shows the provider's attentiveness and sets a reassuring tone.

Common phrases used to ask about comfort:

- *¿Está cómodo(a)?* — Are you comfortable?
- *¿Le duele algo en este momento?* — Is anything hurting right now?
- *¿Necesita que le arregle/acomode la almohada o la manta?* — Would you like me to adjust your pillow or blanket?
- *¿Desea sentarse o acostarse?* — Would you like to sit or lie down?

These types of questions, though seemingly minor, help reduce patient stress and demonstrate empathy.

### 2  Offering Reassurance and Support

Many patients—especially those with limited English proficiency—may feel overwhelmed or uncertain in medical environments. Unfamiliar settings, complex medical terminology, and cultural differences can increase anxiety and reduce patients' willingness to ask questions or express concerns.

Using simple, compassionate statements—such as *"Está en buenas manos"* (You're in good hands), or *"Estamos aquí para ayudarle"* (We're here to help you) —can provide much-needed reassurance and help patients feel more at ease.

Some common examples:

- *Estoy aquí para ayudarle.* — I'm here to help you.
- *No se preocupe, vamos a cuidarle bien.* — Don't worry, we're going to take good care of you.
- *Le explicaré todo paso a paso.* — I will explain everything step by step.
- *Si no entiende algo, por favor pregúnteme / Si algo no le queda claro, por favor pregúnteme.* — If there is anything you don't understand, please ask me.

Using calm and supportive language puts patients at ease and communicates professional confidence.

For many Latinos, family is a central source of emotional and practical support. When clinically appropriate, involving family members can be highly beneficial, especially for patients who may face language barriers.

### 3  Encouraging Openness and Communication

Patients may hesitate to voice discomfort, especially if they feel they are being a burden. Encouraging them to speak openly is essential for safe and effective care.

Useful Examples:

- *Puede decirme si algo le molesta.* — You can tell me if anything bothers you.
- *Avíseme si siente dolor o incomodidad.* — Let me know if you feel pain or discomfort.
- *Su opinión es importante.* — Your opinion is important.
- *¿Tiene alguna pregunta o inquietud?* — Do you have any questions or concerns?

Creating this open channel of communication empowers patients and helps providers better address their needs.

### 4  Building Rapport Through Active Listening and Respect

Rapport extends beyond words. Eye contact, attentive listening, appropriate touch (when culturally accepted), and a calm presence are all tools providers can use to build trust. In addition, understanding nonverbal cues and responding appropriately enhances mutual respect.

Examples of respectful behaviors include:

- Addressing the patient by their preferred name or title.
- Avoiding rushed or abrupt conversation.
- Checking understanding regularly (e.g., *¿Me entiende?* — Do you understand me?; *hasta aquí, ¿tiene alguna duda?* — Any questions so far?).

A brief introduction can go a long way. It helps the patient feel acknowledged, accompanied, and in good hands. Even small moments of clarity can strengthen trust and ease anxiety.

## 2.4 Explaining the Purpose of the Encounter

Explaining why a patient is here is key to good care. In any clinical setting, patients deserve to understand why they are being seen, what the process will involve, and what they can expect throughout the encounter. For Spanish-speaking patients—especially those with limited English proficiency—this clarity is essential to reduce anxiety, foster cooperation, and support informed decision-making.

In Spanish-speaking cultures, where formality, respect, and context matter, explaining the reason for the encounter helps patients feel included and respected in their care journey.

### 1 Setting the Stage with a Clear Introduction

Opening a clinical encounter with a simple explanation of your role and purpose builds trust and helps orient the patient to the process.

Possible phrasing:

- *Estoy aquí para hacerle unas preguntas sobre su salud.* — I'm here to ask you some questions about your health.
- *Soy el médico de turno y quiero conocer su situación.* — I'm the attending physician and I would like to learn about your situation.
- *Soy la enfermera encargada de su evaluación inicial.* — I'm the nurse responsible for your initial assessment.

These statements frame the conversation and set a collaborative tone for what follows.

### 2 Describing the Focus of the Visit

Letting the patient know what will be discussed during the visit allows them to prepare mentally and emotionally. It also helps streamline the interaction by clarifying your intentions.

Model phrases:

- *Vamos a hablar sobre los síntomas que tiene.* — We're going to talk about the symptoms you have.

- *Me gustaría saber más sobre lo que ha estado sintiendo.* — I'd like to know more about what you've been feeling.
- *También revisaremos sus antecedentes médicos.* — We'll also review your medical history.

When patients understand that the provider is actively listening and investigating their condition, they are more likely to share essential information.

### 3  Explaining What Comes Next

Providing an overview of the structure of the visit—even if brief—helps patients feel more comfortable and in control. It also builds confidence in the clinical process.

Model phrases:

- *Le explicaré los próximos pasos / Le voy a explicar qué sigue.* — Let me explain what's next.
- *Le haré un examen físico para evaluar su condición.* — I will perform a physical exam to assess your condition.
- *Si es necesario, pediremos algunos estudios o análisis.* — If necessary, we'll order some tests or lab work.

### 4  Expressing Empathy and Intent to Understand

Healthcare encounters are often stressful. Expressing your intention to understand and help communicate empathy and builds rapport.

Sample phrases:

- *Quiero entender mejor lo que está sintiendo.* — I want to better understand what you're feeling.
- *Estoy aquí para escucharle y ayudarle.* — I'm here to listen and help you.
- *Su bienestar es importante para nosotros.* — Your well-being is important to us.

These affirming messages help reduce emotional barriers and encourage openness.

## 2.5 Basic Questions About Symptoms and Well-being

Initiating a clinical conversation with open-ended, respectful questions is a cornerstone of effective medical communication. In the context of Spanish-speaking patients, asking about symptoms and well-being in a culturally sensitive and linguistically accurate way allows healthcare providers to gather essential clinical information while simultaneously building rapport and trust.

Understanding a patient's current condition begins with clear, empathetic inquiry. Basic questions about symptoms provide critical insight into the nature, duration, and severity of a patient's complaints, and set the stage for deeper diagnostic exploration.

**1** **Starting with Broad, Open-Ended Questions**

Open-ended questions invite the patient to describe their experience in their own words. These types of questions are especially important during the initial portion of the medical interview, as they allow patients to express their concerns freely without feeling rushed or restricted.

You might say:

- *¿Qué le trae hoy a la clínica?* — What brings you to the clinic today?
- *¿Cómo se siente hoy?* — How are you feeling today?
- *¿Le puedo hacer unas preguntas?* — May I ask you a few questions?
- *¿Qué síntomas ha notado últimamente?* — What symptoms have you noticed lately?
- *¿Qué le preocupa más en este momento?* — What concerns you the most right now?
- *Voy a examinarlo(a) ahora, si está bien para usted.* — I'm going to examine you now, if that's okay with you.

These questions demonstrate attentiveness and give providers a comprehensive view of the patient's condition.

**2** **Asking About Pain or Discomfort**

Pain is one of the most common reasons patients seek care. Providers must use clear and compassionate language to inquire about its presence, intensity, and characteristics.

Sample questions for gathering information:

- *¿Siente o tiene algún dolor o molestia?* — Do you have any pain or discomfort?
- *¿Desde hace cuánto tiene el dolor o la molestia?* — Since when have you been experiencing the pain or discomfort?
- *¿Dónde le duele?* — Where does it hurt?
- *¿Cómo describiría el dolor: agudo, sordo, punzante?* — How would you describe the pain: sharp, dull, stabbing?
- *¿El dolor es constante o intermitente?* — Is the pain constant or intermittent?
- *En una escala del 1 al 10, ¿qué tan intenso es el dolor?* — On a scale from 1 to 10, how intense is the pain?
- *¿El dolor se le va a otra parte?* — Does the pain spread to another part of your body?

Understanding the patient's perception of pain is essential for diagnosis and appropriate treatment planning.

**3** **Exploring the Duration and Evolution of Symptoms**

The timeline of symptoms offers valuable diagnostic clues. Providers must be able to inquire about the onset, progression, and resolution of symptoms in clear, chronological terms. Being specific about time and change helps clarify the clinical picture.

Sample questions for gathering information:

- ⊙ *¿Desde cuándo tiene estos síntomas?* — Since when have you had these symptoms?
- ⊙ *¿Cuándo comenzaron exactamente?* — When did they begin exactly?
- ⊙ *¿Han empeorado o mejorado?* — Have they gotten worse or improved?
- ⊙ *¿Qué mejora o empeora el dolor?* — Is there anything that makes the pain feel better or worse?
- ⊙ *¿Los síntomas son iguales todos los días?* — Are the symptoms the same every day?

**4** **Assessing Overall Well-being**

Beyond specific symptoms, it's important to understand how the patient feels in general physically, emotionally, and functionally.

Appropriate wording:

- ⊙ *¿Ha notado algún cambio en su apetito o energía?* — Have you noticed any change in your appetite or energy?
- ⊙ *¿Ha tenido fiebre, escalofríos o sudoración nocturna?* — Have you had fever, chills, or night sweats?
- ⊙ *¿Cómo duerme por las noches?* — How do you sleep at night?

## 2.6 Practical Exercise: Basic Questions in Spanish

Below, you will find a table with an exercise based on a Spanish-speaking patient attending a medical consultation for the first time. In the left column, you will read the dialogue in Spanish, and in the right column, its English translation. Try to identify key phrases in Spanish and compare them with the expressions listed at the end of the table.

| Caso Clínico | Clinical Case |
|---|---|

| Ejemplo de caso en la consulta | Example of a Consultation Case |
|---|---|
| Paciente: Señora García, una mujer de 45 años que acude a la consulta médica por primera vez.<br>Motivo de consulta: Dolor abdominal recurrente y fatiga.<br>Historia clínica: La señora García ha estado experimentando dolor abdominal intermitente durante los últimos 3 meses, acompañado de fatiga y pérdida de apetito. Ha notado que los síntomas empeoran después de comer. | Patient: Mrs. García, a 45-year-old woman who is visiting the medical office for the first time.<br>Chief complaint: Recurrent abdominal pain and fatigue.<br>Medical history: Mrs. García has been experiencing intermittent abdominal pain for the past three months, accompanied by fatigue and loss of appetite. She has noticed that the symptoms worsen after eating. |

| Encuentro inicial | Initial Encounter |
|---|---|
| Médico: "Buenos días, señora García. Gracias por venir a la consulta hoy. ¿Podría contarme un poco más sobre lo que la ha traído aquí? ¿Qué ha estado sintiendo?" | Doctor: "Good morning, Mrs. García. Thank you for coming in today. Could you tell me a little more about what brought you here? What have you been feeling?" |
| Médico: "¿Ha notado algún patrón en relación con el dolor? ¿Algo que lo empeore o lo mejore?" | Doctor: "Have you noticed any pattern related to the pain? Anything that makes it worse or better?" |
| Paciente: "Sí, como mencioné, empeora después de comer. Pero no he notado nada específico que lo mejore." | Patient: "Yes, as I mentioned, it gets worse after eating. But I haven't noticed anything specific that makes it better." |

**Essential Phrases Used During the Initial Encounter.**

1. *Buenos días, gracias por venir a la consulta hoy.* – Good morning, thank you for coming to the appointment today – Warm greeting to establish a positive relationship.

2. *¿Podría contarme un poco más sobre lo que la ha traído aquí?* – Could you tell me a little more about what brought you here? – Open-ended question to obtain detailed information about the symptoms.

3. *¿Qué ha estado sintiendo?* – What have you been feeling? – Follow-up question to deepen understanding of the symptoms.

4. *Entiendo que debe ser muy incómodo para usted.* – I understand this must be very uncomfortable for you. – Empathetic phrase that shows understanding and support.

5. *¿Podría describirme el dolor?* – Could you describe the pain? – Specific question to obtain details about the pain.

6. *¿Ha notado algún patrón en relación con el dolor?* – Have you noticed any pattern related to the pain? – Question aimed at identifying what might trigger or relieve the symptoms.

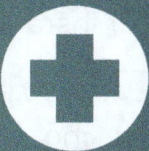

## CHAPTER 3

# UNDERSTANDING PATIENT HISTORY AND SYMPTOMS

## 3.1 Asking About Past Medical History and Conditions

Understanding a patient's past medical history is a cornerstone of safe, personalized, and effective healthcare. This information provides the foundation of the clinical interview and plays a critical role in influencing diagnoses, identifying risk factors, and guiding treatment decisions. For Spanish-speaking patients, the ability to share their medical history in their native language is not only a matter of comfort but also essential to safety and cultural respect. Facilitating this exchange fosters mutual trust and enhances the accuracy of medical care.

### 1 Chronic Illnesses and Long-Term Conditions

Chronic conditions such as diabetes, High Blood Pressure, asthma, and cardiovascular disease require long-term management and can greatly influence the presentation of acute symptoms. Obtaining an accurate history of these conditions enables clinicians to tailor treatment plans and anticipate complications.

Example Questions:

- *¿Tiene antecedentes de enfermedades crónicas como diabetes o hipertensión?* — Do you have a history of chronic illnesses such as diabetes or high blood pressure?

- *¿Tiene algún problema con el corazón, los pulmones, los riñones o el hígado?* — Do you have any problems with your heart, lungs, kidneys, or liver?

### 2 Hospitalizations and Inpatient History

Understanding a patient's history of hospitalization reveals key health events that may not be evident in the current complaint. Questions about past admissions can reveal patterns of care, diagnoses, and emergency interventions.

For instance:

- *¿Ha sido hospitalizado(a) alguna vez? ¿Cuándo y por qué?* — Have you ever been hospitalized? When and why?
- *¿Cuánto tiempo estuvo en el hospital?* — How long were you in the hospital?
- *¿Recibió algún tratamiento especial durante esa hospitalización?* — Did you receive any special treatment during that hospitalization?

### 3  Surgical History

Surgical history is often essential to understanding the root of symptoms or guiding future treatment. Patients may not recall or consider some surgeries relevant, making it important to ask directly about specific procedures and complications.

Try using this:

- *¿Ha tenido alguna cirugía importante?* — Have you had any major surgeries?
- *¿Qué tipo de cirugía fue y en qué año la tuvo?* — What type of surgery was it and in what year?
- *¿Tuvo alguna complicación después de la cirugía?* — Did you have any complications after the surgery?
- *¿Cuántas cesáreas ha tenido? ¿Y, hace cuánto fue la última?* — How many C-sections have you had, and how long ago was the last one?
- *¿Le han realizado cirugía de vesícula (colecistectomía)?* — Have you had gallbladder surgery (cholecystectomy)?

### 4  Family Medical History

Family history is a vital element of preventive care, helping to identify genetic predispositions and informing screening protocols. Asking about diseases in parents, siblings, and extended families can support early intervention and long-term health planning.

Try using this:

- *¿Algún miembro de su familia ha tenido alguna enfermedad importante o crónica?* — Has any family member had a serious or chronic illness?
- *¿Hay antecedentes de cáncer, diabetes o hipertensión... en su familia?* — Is there a family history of cancer, diabetes or high blood pressure...?

Understanding a patient's family history isn't just good medicine — it's a key part of seeing the whole person.

## 3.2 Describing Pain: Location, Type, Intensity

Pain is one of the most common reasons patients seek medical care. Its highly subjective nature makes clear and accurate communication essential for effective diagnosis, treatment, and ongoing management. In Spanish-speaking healthcare interactions, assessing pain involves not only linguistic fluency but also cultural sensitivity and an empathetic approach.

Healthcare professionals must gather detailed information regarding the location, type, intensity, origin, radiation, character, duration, and contributing or relieving factors of pain. Doing so enables clinicians to distinguish between potential causes and tailor care to the patient's unique needs. This chapter provides the essential vocabulary, questions, and cultural considerations for conducting a comprehensive pain assessment in Spanish.

Cultural background significantly influences how patients perceive, express, and respond to pain. In some cultures, expressing pain openly is considered a sign of weakness, leading patients to underreport their symptoms. In others, vocalizing discomfort is seen as a normal and acceptable part of seeking care. Healthcare professionals must remain aware of these variations and avoid making assumptions based solely on visible pain behaviors. Creating a safe and respectful environment encourages honest communication and improves pain management outcomes across diverse populations.

### 1  Asking About the Origen and Location of Pain

Identifying the exact location of pain is the cornerstone of a focused physical examination. Accurate localization can narrow the differential diagnosis and guide the next steps in evaluation.

Phrasing options:

- *¿Dónde le duele?* — Where does it hurt?
- *¿Qué le ocasionó el dolor?* — What caused the pain?
- *¿Puede señalar con el dedo dónde siente el dolor?* — Can you point with your finger to where the pain is?
- *¿Es un dolor profundo o superficial?* — Is it deep or superficial pain?

Taking time to listen carefully and allowing patients to describe their discomfort in detail enhances the quality of the assessment.

### 2  Describing the Type and Quality of Pain

The character or quality of pain can provide important diagnostic clues. Descriptive language helps differentiate between types of pain such as neuropathic, inflammatory, or musculoskeletal.

Effective phrasing:

- *¿Es un dolor agudo, punzante, quemante o sordo?* — Is it sharp, stabbing, burning, or dull pain?
- *¿El dolor se siente como una presión, una punzada o un calambre?* — Does it feel like pressure, a jab, or a cramp?

### 3  Asking About Radiation and Spread

Pain that radiates to other areas of the body can indicate serious underlying conditions, such as cardiac, neurologic, or gastrointestinal disorders. Understanding the pattern of spread is essential for early detection and intervention.

Phrasing options:

- *¿El dolor se queda en un lugar o se irradia a otra parte del cuerpo?* — Does the pain stay in one place or radiate to another part of the body?
- *¿Hacia dónde se extiende el dolor?* — Where does the pain spread?
- *¿Comenzó en un lugar y luego se movió a otro?* — Did it start in one place and move to another?
- *¿Siente el dolor en los brazos, las piernas, el pecho o la espalda?* — Do you feel the pain in your arms, legs, chest, or back?

### 4  Measuring the Intensity of Pain

Measuring pain intensity helps providers track changes, evaluate treatment effectiveness, and adjust therapeutic plans. Using both numerical scales and functional assessments gives a fuller picture of how pain affects daily life.

The following table presents the Visual Analog Scale (VAS) scores, with values ranging from 0 to 10. Additionally, an infographic is provided to help communicate these concepts to children who are not yet able to read.

## Visual Analog Scale (EVA / VAS)[3]

### Escala Visual Análoga del Dolor (EVA)

0 – Sin dolor

1 – Dolor muy leve

2 – Dolor leve

3 – Dolor moderado

4 – Dolor algo fuerte

5 – Dolor fuerte

6 – Dolor muy fuerte

7 – Dolor intenso

8 – Dolor insoportable

9 – Casi el peor dolor imaginable

10 – El peor dolor que pueda imaginar

### Visual Analog Scale (VAS)

0 – No pain

1 – Very mild pain

2 – Mild pain

3 – Moderate pain

4 – Moderately strong pain

5 – Strong pain

6 – Very strong pain

7 – Intense pain

8 – Unbearable pain

9 – Almost the worst imaginable pain

10 – The worst pain imaginable

## ESCALA DE MEDIDOR DE DOLOR

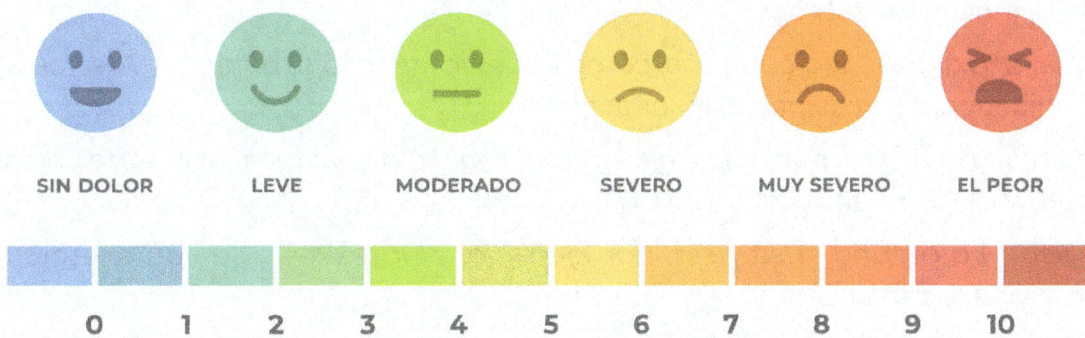

| SIN DOLOR | LEVE | MODERADO | SEVERO | MUY SEVERO | EL PEOR |

0 1 2 3 4 5 6 7 8 9 10

You might say:

- *¿Qué tan fuerte es el dolor del uno al diez? siendo uno sin dolor y diez el peor dolor que pueda imaginar* — How strong is the pain from one to ten? with one being no pain and ten being the worst pain imaginable.

- *¿El dolor le impide dormir o caminar?* — Does the pain prevent you from sleeping or walking?

- *¿Ha tomado algo para aliviar el dolor?* — Have you taken anything to relieve the pain?

Pain intensity scales, along with functional questions, allow clinicians to create more effective and patient-centered treatment plans.

## 3.3 Asking About Allergies and Medications

Ensuring accurate medication information is a foundational responsibility in every healthcare encounter. Understanding a patient's allergies and current medications is essential for preventing adverse drug reactions, ensuring safe prescribing, and promoting positive clinical outcomes. In Spanish-speaking patient interactions, language access is critical to achieving this clarity and ensuring patient safety.

In this section, healthcare professionals will learn how to ask about allergies and medications in clear, respectful Spanish. These conversations should be approached with precision and empathy, especially when patients may not know medical terminology or may have difficulty recalling all the medications they take.

### 1 Asking About Allergies: Critical Safety Information

A detailed allergy history can prevent serious and even life-threatening reactions. Allergies may involve medications, foods, environmental triggers, or materials such as latex. Differentiating between true allergies and side effects is crucial for appropriate medical decision-making.

These are some common ways to ask for it

- *¿Es alérgico(a) a algún medicamento, alimento o sustancia?* — Are you allergic to any medication, food, or substance?

- *¿Es alérgico(a) a algún medicamento, como la penicilina o la aspirina?* — Are you allergic to any medication, such as penicillin or aspirin?

- *¿Es alérgico(a) a algún alimento, por ejemplo, al maní o a los mariscos?* — Are you allergic to any food, such as peanuts or shellfish?

- *¿Es alérgico(a) a alguna sustancia, por ejemplo, al látex?* — Are you allergic to any substance, for example latex?

- *¿Qué tipo de reacción tuvo? ¿Fue leve o grave?* — What kind of reaction did you have? Was it mild or severe?

- *¿Cuándo ocurrió la última reacción?* — When did the last reaction occur?

Asking follow-up questions ensures that the provider correctly distinguishes between allergies and other reactions, guiding safe prescribing practices.

### 2 Asking About Current Medications: Ensuring Continuity of Care

Many patients take a combination of prescription medications, over-the-counter drugs, and dietary supplements. Obtaining an accurate and comprehensive medication list is vital to avoiding harmful interactions and duplications.

Phrasing options:

- *¿Está tomando algún medicamento actualmente?* — Are you currently taking any medications?

- *¿Puede decirme el nombre del medicamento?* — Can you tell me the name of the medication?

- *¿Sabe la dosis y con qué frecuencia lo toma?* — Do you know the dose and how often you take it?

- *¿Lo toma todos los días o solo cuando lo necesita?* — Do you take it every day or only as needed?

If patients are unsure, encourage them to bring a medication list or the medication containers during the next visit.

**3** **Inquiring About Non-Prescription and Herbal Products**

Patients may use herbal remedies, traditional medicine, or non-prescription products that could interfere with prescribed treatments. Asking about these with respect and cultural awareness helps ensure safety while valuing the patient's beliefs.

Some common ways to say this are:

- *¿Toma vitaminas, suplementos o remedios naturales?* — Do you take vitamins, supplements, or natural remedies?

- *¿Usa hierbas medicinales o productos comprados sin receta? ¿Cuáles?* — Do you use medicinal herbs or over-the-counter products? Which ones?

- *¿Ha recibido tratamientos alternativos recientemente? ¿Cuáles?* — Have you received any alternative treatments recently? Which ones?

- *¿Ha notado algún efecto o cambio en su salud desde que empezó a usarlos?* — Have you noticed any effects or changes in your health since you started using them?

Understanding the full range of substances a patient consumes supports a more comprehensive and integrative care approach.

**4** **Reinforcing the Importance of Medication Review**

Explaining the reason for asking about medications and allergies can improve communication and increase cooperation. When patients understand the safety goals behind these questions, they are more likely to participate fully and accurately.

Helpful Phrases:

- *Esta información es importante para evitar efectos secundarios.* — This information is important to avoid side effects.

- *Quiero asegurarme de que los medicamentos sean seguros para usted.* — I want to ensure the medications are safe for you.

- *Gracias por compartir esta información.* — Thank you for sharing this information.

## 3.4 Gathering Social History Relevant to Health

A patient's overall health is influenced not only by biological and clinical conditions, but also by social, behavioral, and environmental circumstances.

Collecting a respectful and detailed social history is an essential part of the clinical interview, offering key insights into the daily factors that influence patient well-being, treatment adherence, and healthcare outcomes.

In Spanish-speaking encounters, it is particularly important to approach these discussions with cultural sensitivity. Many patients may not be accustomed to sharing personal details with healthcare providers. Asking questions in a clear, respectful, and nonjudgmental manner builds trust and promotes openness.

### 1 Tobacco Use: A Key Risk Factor

Tobacco use remains a leading contributor to preventable disease and death. Understanding a patient's smoking habits is foundational for both diagnosis and preventive counseling.

Model phrases:

- *¿Fuma o ha fumado en el pasado?* — Do you smoke, or have you smoked in the past?
- *¿Cuántos cigarrillos fuma al día?* — How many cigarettes do you smoke per day?
- *¿Cuándo comenzó a fumar?* — When did you start smoking?
- *¿Ha considerado dejar de fumar?* — Have you considered quitting smoking?
- *¿Alguna de las personas con las que convive fuma?* — Does anyone you live with smoke?

These questions guide counseling efforts and connect patients to smoking cessation resources.

### 2 Alcohol Use: Exploring Frequency and Quantity

Alcohol use, even at moderate levels, may impact physical and mental health, interfere with medications, and contribute to chronic conditions. Building trust is crucial to obtaining an honest and complete account.

How to word it:

- *¿Consume bebidas alcohólicas? ¿Con qué frecuencia? ¿En qué cantidad?* — Do you consume alcoholic beverages? How often? In what quantity?
- *¿Cuándo empezó a tomar alcohol?* — When did you start drinking alcohol?
- *¿Normalmente qué tipo de bebidas consume?* — What type of drinks do you usually have?
- *¿Cuántos tragos consume en un día típico?* — How many drinks do you have on a typical day?
- *¿Ha tenido problemas relacionados con el alcohol?* — Have you had any problems related to alcohol?

## 3 Drug Use and Substance Exposure

Understanding recreational and non-prescription drug use is vital to assessing health risks and planning treatment. Approaching these questions with tact and compassion encourages openness and supports recovery when needed.

**Cultural Note[1]:** In many Spanish-speaking countries, especially in Latin America, the word "drug(s)" ["droga(s)"] is commonly associated with illicit substances or "hard drugs," rather than prescription medication. Although the World Health Organization (WHO) defines "drug" in pharmacology as any active pharmaceutical ingredient, in everyday language the term often evokes illegal drug use.

For this reason, international health organizations emphasize the importance of using precise, non-stigmatizing terminology when referring to substance use disorders. They recommend phrases such as "person with a substance use disorder" rather than simply "drug user," in order to avoid negative connotations and reduce stigma. Several academic and anthropological studies have documented the cultural sensitivity surrounding the term "droga." In local contexts, it often carries associations with criminality, addiction, or drug trafficking, rather than with clinical or therapeutic use.

Example Questions:

- *¿Consume alguna droga recreativa o sustancias ilegales?* — Do you use any recreational drugs or illegal substances?

- *¿Ha consumido marihuana, cocaína, o medicamentos sin receta (prescripción)?* — Have you used marijuana, cocaine, or medications without a prescription?

- *¿Ha consumido alguna vez sustancias como heroína, metanfetaminas, fentanilo u opiáceos sin receta?* — Have you ever used substances such as heroin, methamphetamines, fentanyl or non-prescribed opioids?

- *¿Ha consumido alguna sustancia alucinógena, como peyote, hongos alucinógenos o LSD?* — Have you ever used any hallucinogenic substances, such as peyote, magic mushrooms, or LSD?

- *¿Con qué frecuencia las ha consumido en los últimos tres meses?* — How often have you used them in the past three months?

- *¿Ha tenido alguna adicción o ha buscado tratamiento por ella?* — Have you ever had any addiction or sought treatment for one?

- *¿Le gustaría hablar con un consejero o especialista en adicciones?* — Would you like to speak with a counselor or addiction specialist?

**4**  **Living Situation and Social Support**

A patient's living environment and support network significantly impact their health and recovery. Identifying barriers to care such as isolation, lack of transportation, or absence of caregivers is critical in care planning.

For instance, you would use:

- *¿Con quién vive? ¿Hay alguien en casa que lo(a) pueda ayudar o acompañar?* — Who do you live with? Is there anyone at home who can help you or come with you?
- *¿Vive solo(a) o acompañado(a)?* — Do you live alone or with someone?
- *¿Tiene cómo transportarse para asistir a sus citas?* — Do you have a way to get to your appointments?
- *¿Hay alguien que lo(a) pueda cuidar si se enferma?* — Is there someone who can take care of you if you become ill?

Understanding the home environment helps providers coordinate resources and discharge plans.

**5**  **Employment and Occupational Risks**

Employment status and work environment provide insight into financial stability, mental health, and potential exposure to occupational hazards. These questions help shape social and clinical support strategies.

You could say, for instance:

- *¿Tiene trabajo? ¿En qué trabaja?* — Do you work? What kind of work do you do?
- *¿Su trabajo implica esfuerzo físico, estrés constante, o exposición a sustancias (productos) químicas?* — Does your job involve physical labor, stress, or exposure to chemicals?
- *¿Tiene seguro médico a través del trabajo?* — Do you have health insurance through your job?
- *¿Está actualmente buscando empleo?* — Are you currently looking for work?

## 3.5 Practical Exercise

The following is a transcript of a conversation between a Spanish-speaking patient and her doctor during a medical consultation. Try to read the Spanish version **first**. However, an English version translation is provided for reference if needed.

After reading it carefully, you will be presented with a few questions in Spanish. Try to answer them before reading the suggested answers in both Spanish and English. Once completed, you will be guided through a series of follow-up steps to consider for a real consultation.

This exercise is designed to help you understand the importance of taking a thorough medical history and recognizing relevant symptoms and patterns in order to provide effective patient care.

# Clinical Case

| Ejercicio de caso en la consulta | Case scenario in the consultation |
|---|---|
| *Una paciente de 32 años, llamada Sofía, acude a la consulta médica con síntomas de dolor de cabeza y fatiga. A continuación, se proporciona una transcripción de la conversación entre el médico y Sofía.* | A 32-year-old patient named Sofía comes to the medical consultation with symptoms of headache and fatigue.<br>Below is a transcript of the conversation between the doctor and Sofía. |

| Transcripción del diálogo | Transcript of the dialogue |
|---|---|
| *Médico: "Buenos días, Sofía. ¿Podrías contarme sobre lo que te ha traído hoy a consulta?"* | Doctor: "Good morning, Sofía. Could you tell me what brought you in today?" |
| *Sofía: "He tenido dolores de cabeza terribles durante las últimas semanas. Me siento cansada todo el tiempo y no puedo concentrarme en el trabajo."* | Sofia: "I've been having terrible headaches over the past few weeks. I feel tired all the time and I can't concentrate at work." |
| *Médico: "¿Desde hace cuánto tienes estos dolores de cabeza? ¿Son constantes o van y vienen?"* | Doctor: "How long have you had these headaches? Are they constant or do they come and go?" |
| *Sofía: "Han sido intermitentes, pero han estado empeorando últimamente. Creo que comenzaron hace unos 3 meses."* | Sofia: "They've been intermittent, but they've been getting worse lately. I think they started around three months ago." |
| *Médico: "¿Has notado algún patrón en relación con los dolores de cabeza? ¿Algo que los empeore o los mejore?"* | Doctor: "Have you noticed any pattern related to the headaches? Anything that makes them worse or better?" |
| *Sofía: "Sí, parecen empeorar cuando estoy estresada o no duermo bien."* | Sofia: "Yes, they seem to get worse when I'm stressed or don't sleep well." |
| *Ejercicio de caso en la consulta* | Case scenario in the consultation |
| *Médico: "¿Tienes algún historial médico relevante o has tomado algún medicamento recientemente?"* | Doctor: "Do you have any relevant medical history or have you taken any medication recently?" |
| *Sofía: "Tengo antecedentes de migrañas en mi familia. Mi madre y mi hermana las sufren."* | Sofia: "I have a family history of migraines. My mother and my sister both suffer from them." |

**Preguntas**:

1. ¿Cuánto tiempo ha estado Sofía experimentando dolores de cabeza? (Duración de los síntomas)
2. ¿Qué factores parecen desencadenar o agravar los dolores de cabeza de Sofía? (Patrón de los síntomas)
3. ¿Qué antecedente médico relevante menciona Sofía que podría estar relacionado con sus síntomas? (Historial médico relevante)
4. ¿Qué síntomas asociados al dolor de cabeza menciona Sofía? (Síntomas asociados)

## Respuestas / Answer

| Spanish | English |
| --- | --- |
| Ha estado experimentándolos durante las últimas semanas, pero cree que comenzaron hace unos tres meses. | She's been having them over the past few weeks, but she thinks they started about three months ago. |
| Los dolores de cabeza parecen empeorar cuando está estresada o no duerme bien. | The headaches seem to get worse when she is stressed or doesn't sleep well. |
| Sofía menciona antecedentes de migrañas en su familia: su madre y su hermana las padecen. | Sofía mentions a family history of migraines: her mother and sister suffer from them. |
| Además del dolor de cabeza, menciona sentirse cansada todo el tiempo y tener dificultad para concentrarse en el trabajo. | In addition to the headache, she says she feels tired all the time and has trouble concentrating at work. |

## Análisis / Analysis

| Spanish | English |
| --- | --- |
| La duración de los síntomas y los patrones observados pueden ayudar a identificar posibles desencadenantes o causas subyacentes. | The duration of symptoms and the observed patterns may help identify possible triggers or underlying causes |
| El historial médico familiar de migrañas podría sugerir una predisposición genética a ciertos tipos de dolores de cabeza. | A family medical history of migraines may suggest a genetic predisposition to certain types of headaches. |
| Los síntomas asociados como la fatiga y la falta de concentración pueden estar relacionados con los dolores de cabeza o podrían indicar otros problemas subyacentes. | Associated symptoms such as fatigue and difficulty concentrating may be related to the headaches or could indicate other underlying issues. |

**Próximos pasos / Next steps:**

- *Realizar una exploración física y obtener más detalles sobre el historial médico de Sofía.*
- (Perform a physical examination and gather more details about Sofía's medical history)
- *Considerar pruebas diagnósticas adicionales si es necesario.*
- (Consider additional diagnostic tests if necessary)
- *Desarrollar un plan de tratamiento basado en los hallazgos del diagnóstico.*
- (Develop a treatment plan based on the diagnostic findings.)

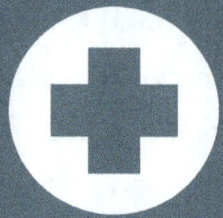

BOOK 3

# PERFORMING THE PHYSICAL EXAM IN SPANISH

## A PRACTICAL GUIDE FOR HEALTHCARE PROVIDERS TO EXPLAIN PROCEDURES AND DOCUMENT PATIENT FINDINGS

ACQUIRE A LOT

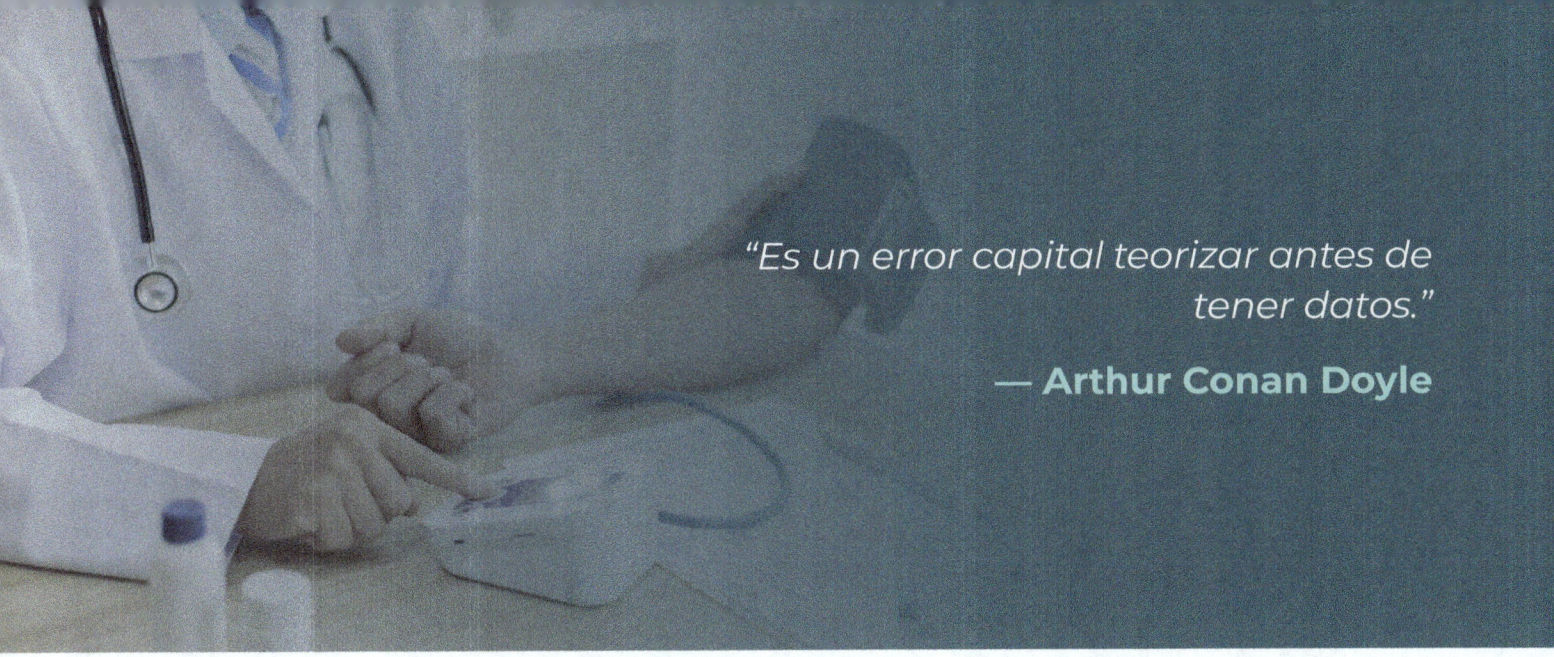

CHAPTER 4

# EXPLAINING EXAMINATION PROCEDURES

## 4.1 Describing Examination Steps: Inspection, Palpation, Percussion, Auscultation

A respectful and detailed explanation of the physical examination fosters trust, cooperation, and understanding — particularly when language or cultural differences are present. Spanish-speaking patients, like all patients, benefit from knowing what to expect.

Explaining each step simply in Spanish ensures precision and respect.

This section focuses on how to introduce the four fundamental techniques used in the physical examination: inspection, palpation, percussion, and auscultation. Each method plays a unique role in the diagnostic process and should be explained with clarity and care.

### 1  *Inspección* (Inspection)

Inspection involves visually examining the patient's body for signs of illness or abnormalities. This may include observing skin color, posture, movement, or the appearance of specific areas.

In Spanish, you could ask:

- ⊙ *Voy a examinar su piel* — I'm going to examine your skin.
- ⊙ *Voy a examinarla / Voy a examinarlo* — I'm going to examine you.
- ⊙ *Voy a examinar sus ojos.* — I'm going to examine your eyes.
- ⊙ *Voy a examinar sus extremidades* — I'm going to check your limbs.

By informing the patient about this non-invasive first step, providers ease anxiety and encourage cooperation.

## 2  *Palpación* (Palpation)

Palpation involves gently touching the body to assess underlying structures, detect tenderness, swelling, or masses, and evaluate temperature or texture. Keep talking clearly and be professional as you go.

Possible phrasing:

- *Voy a tocar suavemente su abdomen para sentir cualquier anomalía.* — I will gently touch your abdomen to feel for any abnormalities.
- *Voy a palpar esta zona para verificar si hay dolor o una masa.* — I'm going to palpate this area to check for pain or a mass.
- *Puede sentir una ligera presión mientras palpo con mis manos. Avíseme si siente molestia o dolor.* — You may feel slight pressure while I palpate with my hands. Let me know if you feel any discomfort or pain.

Always inform the patient before initiating contact and ensure their comfort is maintained.

## 3  *Percusión* (Percussion)

Percussion involves tapping on the body surface to assess the condition of underlying organs and tissues. Different sounds produced during percussion can help diagnose fluid, air, or masses within body cavities.

A common way to say this is:

- *Voy a percutir suavemente su abdomen con mis dedos.* — I'm going to gently percuss your abdomen with my fingers.
- *Voy a percutir ligeramente su tórax con mis dedos.* — I'm going to gently percuss your chest with my fingers.
- *Voy a percutir ligeramente su región lumbar con mis dedos.* — I'm going to gently percuss your lower back with my fingers.

This technique may feel unusual to some patients, so clear explanation and reassurance are helpful.

## 4  *Auscultación* (Auscultation)

Auscultation involves listening to internal body sounds, typically the heart, lungs, and abdomen, using a stethoscope. This technique provides critical information about cardiovascular and respiratory health.

Model phrases you can use:

- *Voy a escuchar su corazón y pulmones con el estetoscopio.* — I'm going to listen to your heart and lungs with the stethoscope.
- *Voy a auscultar su abdomen con el estetoscopio.* — I'm going to auscultate your abdomen with my stethoscope.

In some contexts, you can use the verb "listen" instead of "auscultate". Then the phrase could be:

- *Voy a escuchar su corazón con mi estetoscopio.* — I'm going to listen to your heart with my stethoscope.

Providing a calm and clear explanation helps normalize the experience and maintains professionalism throughout the exam.

Describing each step of the physical examination in Spanish strengthens patient-provider communication, enhances comfort, and promotes understanding. This respectful, transparent approach fosters better clinical outcomes and deepens trust essential elements of patient-centered care.

## 4.2 Giving Instructions for Patient Positioning and Cooperation

Providing clear and respectful instructions on how to move or position the body is vital for an effective and smooth examination.

Clinical Example Phrases:

- *Por favor, siéntese en la camilla.* — Please sit on the examination table.
- *Acuéstese boca arriba.* — Lie on your back.
- *Gire hacia su lado izquierdo.* — Turn to your left side.
- *Respire profundo (profundamente/hondo) y mantenga el aire.* — Take a deep breath and hold it.
- *Relaje los músculos, por favor.* — Please relax your muscles.
- *Por favor, doble su brazo.* — Please bend your arm.
- *Por favor, flexione sus rodillas.* — Please flex your knees.

## 4.3 Explaining the Use of Medical Instruments

Explaining what each medical instrument is and how it will be used is a simple yet powerful way to build trust, reduce anxiety, and create a more collaborative clinical environment. Many patients, especially those who are unfamiliar with medical procedures or who speak a different primary language, may feel nervous or unsure when unfamiliar tools are introduced. In Spanish-speaking encounters, describing each instrument using clear and respectful language helps reassure patients and enhances the overall care experience.

Introducing each tool with a brief explanation of its purpose helps demystify the exam process and makes the interaction more transparent. This step is especially important in pediatrics, geriatrics, and cross-cultural settings, where unfamiliarity with medical instruments may increase anxiety or discomfort.

**Common Medical Instruments and Spanish Phrases**

Use the following phrases to introduce commonly used tools during a physical exam:

- *Este es un estetoscopio; voy a escuchar su corazón / pulmones.* — This is a stethoscope; I'm going to listen to your heart / lungs.

- *Voy a usar este otoscopio para examinar sus oídos.* — I'm going to use this otoscope to examine your ears.

- *Este aparato sirve para medir su presión arterial.* — This device is used to measure your blood pressure.

- *Voy a usar este termómetro para tomar su temperatura.* — I'm going to use this thermometer to take your temperature.

- *Voy a usar este martillo para evaluar sus reflejos.* — I'm going to use this reflex hammer to check your reflexes.

**Best Practices for Introducing Instruments**

1. Show the instrument before using it.
2. Explain what you will do and why.
3. Use simple and reassuring language.
4. Observe the patient's response and offer reassurance if needed.
5. Ask for permission or consent before proceeding.
6. Maintain a calm, professional and respectful demeanor.
7. Ensure the patient's privacy and comfort.
8. Describe what the patient may feel during the procedure.
9. Clean or disinfect the instrument in front of the patient when appropriate.

Taking a moment to introduce medical instruments fosters patient comfort and cooperation. In Spanish-speaking settings, this approach helps bridge communication gaps and supports a relationship built on respect and understanding. Clear, empathetic communication is key to a positive and effective medical experience.

## 4.4 Ensuring Patient Comfort and Addressing Concerns

Patient comfort is not only a marker of good bedside manners, but also essential to the success of any physical examination. Attending a patient's emotional and physical well-being enhances the quality of care, fosters trust, and improves cooperation. When patients feel respected, safe, and heard, they are more likely to communicate openly, follow recommendations, and return for care.

In Spanish-speaking clinical settings, ensuring comfort requires clear communication in the patient's preferred language and a culturally sensitive approach. Patients may hesitate to express discomfort or confusion, so it is the provider's responsibility to proactively check in, offer reassurance, and explain each step of the examination.

## Monitoring Comfort During the Exam

Throughout the physical exam, providers should observe both verbal and non-verbal signs of discomfort. Asking simple, direct questions in Spanish gives patients the opportunity to express how they are feeling and encourages a collaborative tone.

You might say:

- *¿Está cómodo(a)? ¿Siente dolor?* — Are you comfortable? Do you feel any pain?
- *Si algo le incomoda, por favor dígamelo.* — If anything bothers you, please let me know.

## Ending Each Phase of the Exam Respectfully

Concluding each portion of the exam with acknowledgment and thanks reinforces patient dignity. It signals respect for their participation and builds rapport for future interactions.

A common way to say this is:

- *Ya terminamos con esta parte. Gracias por su cooperación.* — We're done with this part. Thank you for your cooperation.

## Addressing Questions and Concerns

Make an effort to provide space for questions and acknowledge any patient concerns in a respectful, non-rushed manner. Many Spanish-speaking patients may come from cultural backgrounds where questioning medical authority is uncommon. By explicitly inviting dialogue, providers empower patients to voice their needs.

Try using this:

- *¿Tiene alguna pregunta o inquietud?* — Do you have any questions or concerns?
- *Estoy aquí para ayudarle.* — I'm here to help you.

By proactively monitoring comfort and encouraging communication, healthcare professionals create a more humane and effective clinical environment. These small steps show patients they're part of the team and improve care.

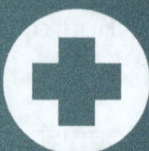

## CHAPTER 5

# DESCRIBING PHYSICAL EXAMINATION FINDINGS

### 5.1 General Appearance and Vital Signs

The initial impression of a patient's general appearance, combined with their vital signs, provides critical context for the entire clinical assessment. These observations are among the first pieces of data gathered during the physical exam and often set the stage for subsequent evaluations. In Spanish-speaking healthcare settings, communicating these findings clearly and accurately helps maintain transparency and strengthens the provider-patient relationship.

Documenting general appearance involves assessing the patient's level of alertness, distress, hygiene, and overall physical condition. Vital signs—such as blood pressure, heart rate, respiratory rate, and temperature—are objective measures of physiological status. Together, they offer a snapshot of the patient's immediate health and guide medical decision-making.

**1  General Appearance**

A provider's description of general appearance is based on visual and behavioral observations. These observations can reveal underlying illness or distress even before vital signs are obtained.

Possible phrasing:

- *El paciente parece alerta y en buen estado general.* — The patient appears alert and in generally good condition.

Other useful descriptors may include terms for fatigue, discomfort, pallor, or confusion. This qualitative assessment complements quantitative data collected later in the exam.

**2  Recording Vital Signs**

Vital signs are fundamental indicators of a patient's health and are measured routinely during physical examinations. Accurate collection and documentation are essential to monitor changes, detect instability, and guide treatment.

Common examples:

- *Presión arterial: 120 sobre 80.* — Blood pressure: 120 over 80.
- *Temperatura, frecuencia cardíaca, frecuencia respiratoria: normales.* — Temperature, heart rate, and respiratory rate: normal.
- *Frecuencia cardíaca: 72 latidos por minuto.* — Heart rate: 72 beats per minute.
- *Temperatura corporal: 37 grados Celsius.* — Body temperature: 37 degrees Celsius.

Note that most Spanish-speaking countries use the metric system, as opposed to the imperial system commonly used in the United States. As a result, measurements for weight, length, area, and temperature may appear in units different from those typically used in English-speaking healthcare settings. This distinction is especially important when reviewing medical records or interacting with patients who may not be familiar with the units used in your facility.

### 3 Communicating Vital Signs to the Patient

While vital signs are typically documented for clinical use, sharing the information with the patient, especially in their native language, helps reinforce engagement in their own care. It can also provide reassurance or prompt further discussion when abnormalities are found.

In Spanish, you could say:

- *Su presión arterial está dentro del rango normal.* — Your blood pressure is within the normal range.
- *Su temperatura es normal.* — Your temperature is normal.
- *Vamos a monitorear regularmente sus signos vitales.* — We're going to monitor your vital signs regularly.

Observing general appearance and recording vital signs may seem routine, but they are fundamental to every physical examination. These initial assessments provide vital insights and set the tone for the clinical encounter. In Spanish-speaking settings, explaining this process clearly and respectfully supports patient understanding and promotes collaborative care.

## 5.2 Cardiovascular Examination: Heart Sounds and Pulses

Cardiovascular examination is a critical component of physical assessment. It provides essential insights into the health of the heart and vascular system. Observations should be detailed and systematic, focusing on heart rhythm, audible sounds such as murmurs, and the presence and quality of peripheral pulses. These elements help detect conditions ranging from arrhythmias to vascular insufficiencies.

In Spanish-speaking healthcare settings, describing cardiovascular findings in a clear and professional manner both in clinical documentation and in patient communication enhances care quality and strengthens trust between provider and patient.

## 1 Heart Sounds and Rhythm

Auscultation of the heart allows the clinician to assess the rate, rhythm, and to detect any abnormal sounds such as murmurs, clicks, or gallops. A regular rhythm and absence of murmurs are typical of a healthy cardiac exam.

Appropriate wording:

- *Ritmo cardíaco regular, sin soplos.* — Regular heart rhythm, no murmurs.
- *El paciente presenta un ritmo cardíaco irregular. Es necesario estudiar más a fondo la causa de esta arritmia.* — The patient has an irregular heart rhythm. It is necessary to investigate the cause of this arrhythmia further.
- *Tiene un soplo en una parte del corazón llamada válvula mitral. Vamos a hacerle más estudios para comprender mejor qué está ocurriendo* — You have a murmur in a part of your heart called the mitral valve. We'll do more tests to better understand what's going on.

## 2 Peripheral Pulses

Palpation of peripheral pulses helps evaluate vascular perfusion and symmetry. Pulses should be assessed bilaterally at multiple sites, including the radial, femoral, popliteal, posterior tibial, and dorsalis pedis arteries.

Practical everyday expressions:

- *Pulsos periféricos presentes y simétricos.* — Peripheral pulses present and symmetrical.
- *Pulsos ausentes, disminuidos o asimétricos pueden sugerir enfermedad vascular u oclusión, lo que requiere una evaluación adicional.* — Absent, diminished, or asymmetric pulses may suggest vascular disease or occlusion, prompting further investigation.
- *Presenta un pulso débil en las extremidades inferiores.* — There is a weak pulse in the lower extremities.

## 3 Capillary refill

Capillary refill time is a quick bedside test to assess peripheral perfusion. Pressing on a nail bed and observing the time for color to return helps evaluate circulatory status.

You would use this:

- Tiene un llenado capilar normal, menor a 2 segundos — He/She has a normal capillary refill, under 2 seconds.
- *El llenado capilar es anormal en la mano derecha* — Capillary refill is abnormal in the right hand.

## 4 Communicating Findings to the Patient

When appropriate, explain your findings to the patient clearly and reassure. For Spanish-speaking patients, use straightforward language to describe what you are listening for and what the results mean.

A common way to say it is:

- *Estoy escuchando su corazón para revisar el ritmo y los sonidos.* — I'm listening to your heart to check the rhythm and sounds.
- *Sus pulsos se sienten normales y parejos.* — Your pulses feel normal and even.
- *No escucho sonidos anormales en su corazón.* — I don't hear any abnormal sounds in your heart.

The cardiovascular exam is a vital part of evaluating a patient's overall health. Accurate assessment of heart sounds and peripheral pulses provides essential diagnostic information and helps detect potentially serious conditions early. Clear communication in Spanish not only supports high-quality documentation but also empowers patients through transparency and shared understanding.

## 5.3 Abdominal Examination: Bowel Sounds and Palpation

The abdominal examination is a principal part of the physical exam, offering critical insight into the function and condition of the gastrointestinal system. Clinicians assess the abdomen through inspection, auscultation, percussion, and palpation—looking for signs such as tenderness, abnormal bowel sounds, or palpable masses. This structured evaluation helps identify conditions ranging from acute inflammation to bowel obstruction or organomegaly.

For Spanish-speaking patients, explaining the process and findings in their preferred language supports understanding, alleviates anxiety, and strengthens the patient-provider relationship.

### 1 Bowel Sounds

Auscultation of the abdomen involves listening for bowel sounds in all four quadrants. These sounds provide information about intestinal activity and can help detect abnormalities such as obstruction or ileus.

How to document it:

- *Presencia de ruidos intestinales normales en los cuatro cuadrantes.* — Normal bowel sounds in all four quadrants.
- *Ruidos intestinales aumentados.* — Increased bowel sounds.

Absence, decrease, or excessive bowel sounds can be significant, prompting further investigation. Clear documentation is essential for tracking changes and guiding clinical decisions.

### 2 Palpation and Assessment of Tenderness

Palpation is used to evaluate tenderness, guarding, rigidity, and the presence of masses or organ enlargement. This part of the exam should be performed gently and with attention to patient comfort.

Suggested Documentation:

- ⊙ *Abdomen blando, no doloroso a la palpación.* — Soft abdomen, non-tender to palpation.
- ⊙ *Abdomen doloroso, con defensa muscular en el cuadrante inferior derecho.* — Tender abdomen with guarding in the right lower quadrant.

The term *'blando'* (soft) indicates a relaxed abdominal wall, while noting the absence or presence of tenderness helps determine next steps in evaluation or imaging.

### 3 Communicating the Process and Findings

It is important to explain what you are doing and why at each stage of the abdominal exam. This reassurance helps patients feel more at ease and allows for clearer clinical communication in Spanish-speaking interactions.

Model phrases you can use:

- ⊙ *Voy a escuchar su abdomen para revisar los ruidos intestinales.* — I'm going to listen to your abdomen to check the bowel sounds.
- ⊙ *Voy a presionar suavemente en varias áreas para ver si siente dolor.* — I'm going to press gently in several areas to see if you feel any pain.
- ⊙ *Si siente molestias, por favor avíseme.* — Please let me know if you feel any discomfort.

The abdominal exam offers valuable clinical insights that guide diagnosis and treatment decisions. Performing this assessment with precision, empathy, and linguistic clarity—especially with Spanish-speaking patients—ensures a more inclusive and effective healthcare experience. Respectful, informed interaction during the exam reinforces patient trust and enhances the overall quality of care.

## 5.4 Musculoskeletal Examination: Range of Motion and Strength

The musculoskeletal examination plays a vital role in assessing physical function, mobility, and strength. It helps detect conditions affecting muscles, joints, bones, and connective tissue. A complete evaluation includes observing muscle tone, measuring strength, assessing joint range of motion, and evaluating for pain, swelling, or deformity.

In Spanish-speaking clinical settings, clearly communicating each part of the examination ensures patient understanding and encourages cooperation. Describing findings in Spanish also promotes transparency, comfort, and trust—essential aspects of patient-centered care.

### 1 Muscle Strength Assessment

Muscle strength is typically graded on a scale of 0 to 5, with 5 representing normal strength. This part of the exam evaluates the patient's ability to resist force during specific movements. Symmetry and balance between limbs are also noted.

Example Phrases:

- *Fuerza muscular 5/5 en extremidades superiores e inferiores.* — Muscle strength 5/5 in upper and lower limbs.
- *Fuerza muscular 3/5, disminuida en el miembro inferior izquierdo.* — Muscle strength 3/5, decreased in the left lower limb.

These phrases indicate that the patient demonstrates normal or abnormal strength in both the arms and legs, without weakness or asymmetry.

## 2  Joint Range of Motion

Range of motion refers to how far a joint can move in various directions. Full, pain-free range is considered normal. Any limitation, stiffness, or pain should be noted and may require further evaluation through imaging or physical therapy.

Possible phrasing:

- *Arcos de movimiento completos sin dolor.* — Full range of motion without pain.
- *Limitación en los arcos de movimiento del miembro superior derecho, con dolor.* — Painful limitation of range of motion in the right upper extremity.

Clinicians often assess both active and passive movements across multiple joints to identify functional impairments or structural abnormalities.

## 3  Communicating the Exam to the Patient

Effective communication during the musculoskeletal exam ensures that patients are informed and at ease. In Spanish-speaking encounters, providers should describe each maneuver before proceeding and reassure the patient that any discomfort should be reported.

Helpful phrases for clear communication:

- *Voy a evaluar su fuerza muscular en brazos y piernas.* — I'm going to assess your muscle strength in your arms and legs.
- *Por favor, empuje contra mi mano.* — Please push against my hand.
- *Ahora voy a manipular sus articulaciones para revisar su movilidad.* — Now I'm going to move your joints to check your range of motion.
- *Por favor, avíseme si siente dolor o molestia.* — Let me know if you feel pain or discomfort.

The musculoskeletal exam offers essential information about a patient's physical capabilities, comfort, and quality of life. By assessing strength and mobility in a structured and respectful manner—and by communicating clearly in Spanish when needed—providers ensure accurate findings and build meaningful rapport with their patients.

**Clinical Case:**

This clinical case is designed for healthcare professionals learning medical Spanish. It presents a realistic scenario to help you practice clinical vocabulary, reading comprehension, and diagnostic reasoning in Spanish. The questions encourage you to identify and interpret key findings from the physical examination. At the end of the case, you will find an English version of the full text. It is provided only as a content reference to support understanding. You are encouraged to focus on the original Spanish version to strengthen your language proficiency in a real clinical context.

## Presentación

Un paciente de 55 años, llamado Juan, acude a la consulta médica con síntomas de dolor en el pecho y disnea. Después de obtener su historia clínica, el médico procede a realizar una exploración física. A continuación, se describen los hallazgos positivos de ese examen.

## Hallazgos de la exploración física

- Frecuencia cardíaca: 110 latidos por minuto.
- Presión arterial: 140/90 mmHg.
- Frecuencia respiratoria: 24 respiraciones por minuto.
- Temperatura corporal: 37,2°C.
- Saturación de oxígeno (SaO$_2$): 91%
- Auscultación pulmonar: Se escuchan crepitaciones en las bases de ambos pulmones.
- Auscultación cardíaca: Se detecta un soplo sistólico grado 2/6 en el foco aórtico.
- Edema: Se observa edema 2+ (grado II) en los tobillos.

## Instrucciones

Basándose en los hallazgos de la exploración física de Juan, responda las siguientes preguntas:

1. Frecuencia cardíaca: ¿Qué se puede inferir sobre la frecuencia cardíaca de Juan en comparación con los valores normales?

2. Auscultación pulmonar: ¿Qué sugieren las crepitaciones escuchadas en las bases de ambos pulmones?

3. Auscultación cardíaca: ¿Qué podría indicar la presencia de un soplo sistólico en el foco aórtico?

4. Edema: ¿Qué podría sugerir el edema 2+ (grado II) en los tobillos de Juan?

**Respuestas**

1.  La frecuencia cardíaca de Juan está elevada (taquicardia). Esto puede deberse a múltiples causas como dolor, ansiedad, hipoxia o patología cardíaca subyacente (p. ej., insuficiencia cardíaca).

2.  Las crepitaciones basales bilaterales pueden sugerir la presencia de congestión pulmonar, lo que podría estar relacionado con insuficiencia cardíaca, neumonía u otras condiciones pulmonares.

3.  La presencia de un soplo sistólico en el foco aórtico podría indicar una posible estenosis aórtica u otros problemas valvulares, aunque se necesitarían más pruebas para confirmar el diagnóstico.

4.  El edema 2+ (grado II) en los tobillos de Juan podría sugerir retención de líquidos, lo cual es común en condiciones como insuficiencia cardíaca, problemas renales o hepáticos.

**Análisis**

Los hallazgos de la exploración física proporcionan pistas importantes sobre el estado de salud de Juan y pueden guiar las pruebas diagnósticas adicionales y el plan de tratamiento. Es crucial correlacionar estos hallazgos con la historia clínica y los resultados de otras pruebas para obtener un diagnóstico preciso.

**Próximos pasos**

- Solicitar pruebas diagnósticas adicionales como radiografía de tórax, electrocardiograma (ECG) y análisis de sangre.

- Solicitar valoración por cardiología.

- Considerar estudios cardiacos adicionales como ecocardiograma, pruebas funcionales y biomarcadores cardiacos.

- Desarrollar un plan de tratamiento basado en los diagnósticos confirmados.

- **Tenga en cuenta**: Este ejercicio resalta la importancia del examen físico en el proceso diagnóstico y cómo los hallazgos pueden orientar las decisiones clínicas.

**Clinical Case (English Version)**

A 55-year-old patient named Juan comes to the medical consultation with symptoms of chest pain and shortness of breath. After obtaining his medical history, the physician proceeds with a physical examination. The positive findings from this exam are described below.

**Physical Examination Findings**

- Heart rate: 110 beats per minute.

- Blood pressure: 140/90 mmHg.

- Respiratory rate: 24 breaths per minute.

- Body temperature: 37.2° C.

- Oxygen saturation ($SaO_2$): 91%

- Pulmonary auscultation: Crackles are heard at the bases of both lungs.
- Cardiac auscultation: A grade 2/6 systolic murmur is detected at the aortic focus.
- Edema: 2+ (grade II) edema is observed in the ankles.

## Instructions

Based on Juan's physical examination findings, answer the following questions:

1. Heart rate: What can be inferred about Juan's heart rate compared to normal values?
2. Pulmonary auscultation: What do the crackles heard at the lung bases suggest?
3. Cardiac auscultation: What could the presence of a systolic murmur at the aortic focus indicate?
4. Edema: What might the 2+ (grade II) edema in Juan's ankles suggest?

## Answers

1. Juan's heart rate is elevated (tachycardia). This may be due to multiple causes such as pain, anxiety, hypoxia, or underlying cardiac conditions (e.g., heart failure).
2. Bilateral basal crackles may suggest the presence of pulmonary congestion, which could be related to heart failure, pneumonia, or other pulmonary conditions.
3. The presence of a systolic murmur at the aortic focus could indicate possible aortic stenosis or other valvular problems, although further testing would be needed to confirm the diagnosis.
4. The 2+ (grade II) edema in Juan's ankles could suggest fluid retention, which is common in conditions such as heart failure, renal, or hepatic disorders.

## Analysis

The findings from the physical examination provide important clues about Juan's health status and can guide additional diagnostic testing and treatment planning. It is crucial to correlate these findings with the medical history and other test results to arrive at an accurate diagnosis.

## Next Steps

- Request additional diagnostic tests such as chest X-ray, electrocardiogram (ECG), and blood tests.
- Request a cardiology consultation.
- Consider additional cardiac studies such as echocardiogram, functional tests, and cardiac biomarkers.
- Develop a treatment plan based on the confirmed diagnoses.

**Please note**: This exercise highlights the importance of the physical examination in the diagnostic process and how findings can guide clinical decisions.

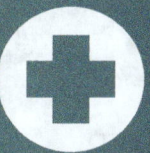

CHAPTER 6

# DOCUMENTING EXAMINATION FINDINGS IN SPANISH

## 6.1 Common Abbreviations and Acronyms in Spanish Medical Notes

Medical documentation relies on clear, standardized language to communicate clinical findings efficiently and accurately. In Spanish-language medical settings, familiarity with common abbreviations and acronyms streamlines note writing, enhances communication among care teams, and ensures consistency in patient records. These abbreviations are frequently used across specialties and healthcare systems to summarize essential clinical information.

Learning and using these standard forms appropriately is a key skill for anyone working in Spanish-speaking medical environments. This section outlines some of the most frequently encountered abbreviations and their English equivalents, helping learners and professionals gain fluency in both language and clinical documentation.

### Common Spanish Abbreviations in Clinical Documentation

Below you will find a list of frequently used abbreviations along with their meanings in Spanish and English.

### Selected Examples of Common Medical Abbreviations

| Abreviatura / Abbreviation | Español / Spanish | English / Inglés |
|---|---|---|
| ECG (EKG) | Electrocardiograma | Electrocardiogram |
| EPOC | Enfermedad Pulmonar Obstructiva Crónica | Chronic Obstructive Pulmonary Disease (COPD) |
| FC | Frecuencia Cardíaca | Heart Rate |

| Abreviatura / Abbreviation | Español / Spanish | English / Inglés |
|---|---|---|
| FR | Frecuencia Respiratoria | Respiratory Rate |
| HTA | Hipertensión Arterial | High Blood Pressure |
| IAM | Infarto Agudo del Miocardio | Acute Myocardial Infarction (AMI) |
| ITU/IVU | Infección del tracto urinario / Infección de vías urinarias | Urinary Tract Infection (UTI) |
| RM | Resonancia Magnética | Magnetic Resonance Imaging (MRI) |
| SaO2 | Saturación Arterial de Oxígeno | Arterial Oxygen Saturation |
| T (T°) | Temperatura | Temperature |
| TA | Tensión Arterial | Blood Pressure |
| TAC | Tomografía Axial Computarizada | Computed Tomography (CT Scan) |

For additional abbreviations, please refer to Chapter 18: Common Medical Abbreviations and Acronyms in Spanish.

**Using Abbreviations Effectively**

While abbreviations enhance efficiency, they must be used thoughtfully. Always consider the clarity of your notes for other healthcare providers and, when necessary, pair abbreviations include with the full form at first mention in any document. This is especially important when communicating across multidisciplinary teams or training environments.

Additionally, avoid non-standard or ambiguous abbreviations that may lead to misunderstandings. When in doubt, clarity should take precedence over brevity.

Mastering common medical abbreviations in Spanish not only improves documentation speed and accuracy but also enhances interprofessional communication and patient safety. As with any aspect of medical language, consistent use and ongoing exposure will strengthen your fluency and confidence in clinical settings.

## 6.2 Describing Normal and Abnormal Findings Using Precise Terminology

Accurate and professional documentation is a cornerstone of effective medical care. When recording examination findings, it is essential to use clear, objective, and nonjudgmental language.

This practice ensures clarity in clinical communication, supports accurate diagnoses, and contributes to continuity of care across medical teams.

In Spanish-language medical records, the use of standardized and precise terminology helps reduce ambiguity and enhances understanding among providers. Whether noting normal observations or describing abnormal signs, the tone should remain neutral and factual. Avoiding subjective interpretations or emotionally charged language ensures that documentation remains professional and useful.

## 1 Documenting Normal Findings

Normal findings should be stated clearly, using terminology that reflects the absence of pathological signs. The phrase *"sin hallazgos anormales"* (no abnormal findings) is commonly used and widely understood in clinical notes. However, it is important that any symptom or clinical sign relevant to the case be described in its normal condition.

Phrasing options:

- *Normal: sin hallazgos anormales* — Normal: no abnormal findings
- *Sistema cardiovascular normal, sin alteraciones evidentes* — Normal cardiovascular system, with no evident abnormalities.
- *Reflejos osteotendinosos normales en miembros inferiores* — Normal deep tendon reflexes in the lower limbs.

These phrases indicate that no clinically significant abnormalities were observed during the examination. It should be used when all relevant systems or areas are assessed and found to be within normal limits.

In certain cases, it is essential to document the absence of symptoms or signs that are relevant to the patient's management or treatment. For example: *Babinski bilateral ausente*—Bilateral Babinski absent. Another example is: *No hay rigidez de nuca*—No nuchal rigidity. Documenting the absence of these clinical signs is essential to ensure that the reader of the medical record is fully informed about the patient's current condition and can accurately interpret the clinical assessment.

## 2 Documenting Abnormal Findings

When abnormal findings are present, they should be described with as much specificity as possible. Use descriptive terms to communicate the type, location, and severity of the condition observed.

Model Phrases for documenting:

- *Anormal: edema leve en extremidades* — Abnormal: mild edema in extremities.
- *Se observa eritema en la zona afectada* — Erythema observed in affected area.

These phrases help convey clinically relevant information without interpretation, as they document observations in an objective manner. Avoid vague terms like 'appears sick' (*"apariencia general enferma"*) or 'seems uncomfortable' (*"con signos de incomodidad"*). Instead, describe what you objectively observe, such as pallor, sweating, grimacing, or restlessness. This ensures clarity and reduces ambiguity in clinical documentation.

### 3 Best Practices for Objective Documentation

- Focus on what you can observe, measure, or verify.
- Use medically accepted terminology and avoid colloquialisms.
- Document findings in a consistent format to support clarity and comparison over time.
- Separate patient-reported symptoms from clinician-observed signs.

Using precise and professional terminology in Spanish medical documentation enhances the quality and reliability of clinical records. Whether describing normal or abnormal findings, clarity and neutrality should always be the goal. This approach not only improves communication among healthcare providers but also upholds the standard of care across language and cultural boundaries.

## 6.3 Documenting Vital Signs and Measurements

Vital signs are fundamental indicators of a patient's physiological state and are among the first metrics recorded during a clinical visit. They offer a rapid assessment of cardiovascular, respiratory, and general metabolic function.

Accurate documentation of these measurements is essential for establishing a baseline, identifying clinical deterioration, and monitoring treatment response.

In Spanish-speaking healthcare settings, the consistent and standardized recording of vital signs supports both effective communication and continuity of care. Proper formatting and terminology ensure that the data is easily understood by all members of the healthcare team.

### 1 Key Vital Signs to Document

The following are the standard vital signs typically recorded during an exam, along with their corresponding Spanish abbreviations and units of measurement:

- *TA: 118/76 mmHg — Tensión arterial (Blood pressure).*
- *FC: 78 lpm — Frecuencia cardíaca (Heart rate, beats per minute).*
- *T: 37.1°C — Temperatura (Body temperature, degrees Celsius).*
- *FR: 16 rpm — Frecuencia respiratoria (Respiratory rate, breaths per minute).*
- *Saturación de oxígeno: 98% — Oxygen saturation.*

### 2 Best Practices for Recording Vital Signs

- Ensure that each measurement is taken using calibrated equipment.
- Record values in the appropriate units (e.g., mmHg, °C, %, lpm). Here is an example of how to record blood pressure: *"Tensión arterial: 159/91 mmHg."*

- Document the time and context of the measurement if relevant (e.g., before medication or post-procedure). For example: *"La tensión arterial se tomó después de que el paciente permaneciera sentado durante 10 minutos."*—Blood pressure was measured after the patient had been seated for 10 minutes.

- If abnormal, note whether the patient is symptomatic and if the value was rechecked. An example of this situation could be: *"El paciente manifestó cefalea durante la toma de la presión arterial, la cual se repitió a los 10 minutos obteniéndose una cifra de 159/85 mmHg."*—The patient reported headache during blood pressure measurement. The reading was repeated after 10 minutes, yielding a value of 159/85 mmHg.

- Use standardized abbreviations to ensure clarity across healthcare teams. Keep in mind that since 2004, The Joint Commission, which accredits hospitals and clinics in the U.S., requires healthcare institutions to maintain a minimum "Do Not Use" list of abbreviations. Always use your institution's approved list of abbreviations, if available. If you must use a lesser-known abbreviation, clearly define its meaning the first time it appears in the documentation.

- Also keep in mind that when reviewing clinical documents written in Spanish, there may not be a standardized use of abbreviations across healthcare professionals. Always verify the meaning of unfamiliar abbreviations using trusted or approved sources.

### 3 Communicating Vital Signs to the Patient

Explaining vital sign readings to patients, especially in their native language, enhances understanding and engagement. This is particularly important when results are outside the normal range or require follow-up care.

How to word it:

- *Su presión arterial está en un rango saludable.* — Your blood pressure is healthy range.

- *Vamos a revisar su temperatura nuevamente más tarde.* — We'll check your temperature again later.

- *Su oxigenación es adecuada en este momento.* — Your oxygen level is adequate at this time.

Vital signs are among the most frequently documented data in clinical care—and among the most significant. Maintaining accuracy, consistency, and clarity in how these values are recorded in Spanish not only ensures high-quality documentation but also supports effective, patient-centered care across language barriers.

## 6.4 Writing Concise and Accurate Examination Reports

A well-written examination report is a cornerstone of professional clinical documentation. It provides a structured, concise summary of the patient's condition and findings from the physical examination. The report should reflect objective observations and avoid unnecessary interpretation or speculation. This format supports continuity of care, clinical decision-making, and effective communication among healthcare providers.

In Spanish-speaking clinical environments, using precise language and standard phrasing ensures clarity and consistency. A clear and professional tone enhances the value of the medical record and helps reduce errors or misinterpretation.

### 1 Key Elements of a Clinical Examination Report

A concise examination report typically includes the following components:

- General condition of the patient
- Significant or notable findings (normal or abnormal)
- Any relevant vitals or observations
- A summary assessment or conclusion.

### 2 Example: Standard Clinical Summary in Spanish

The following is an example of an appropriately phrased clinical summary written in Spanish, accompanied by its English translation. It is part of a series of examples illustrating different ways to summarize a patient's clinical condition, demonstrating variations in tone, structure, and level of detail depending on the context:

- *Paciente en buen estado general, sin signos de alarma, sin evidencias de compromiso agudo. Examen físico sin alteraciones significativas* — Patient in good general condition, with no red flags and no evidence of acute compromise. Physical examination unremarkable.

- *Paciente femenina en condición general estable, con signos vitales dentro de los rangos normales, sin signos de alarma ni indicios de patología aguda. Examen físico sin hallazgos relevantes, sin signos de compromiso localizado ni sistémico.* — Female patient in stable general condition, vital signs within normal range, without red flags or signs of acute pathology. Physical exam unremarkable, with no signs of localized or systemic compromise.

This is a fuller example:

- *Paciente en condición general estable, con signos vitales dentro de los rangos normales. Consulta por seguimiento de condición crónica, sin referir síntomas nuevos ni signos de alarma. Niega fiebre, dolor, disnea u otras manifestaciones clínicas relevantes. Durante la valoración, se encuentra en buen estado general, alerta, orientada, y con adecuado estado nutricional e hidratación. El examen físico se encuentra dentro de los parámetros normales, sin evidencias de compromiso localizado ni sistémico. Se continúa con el manejo habitual, sin necesidad de ajustes en el tratamiento actual, y se recomienda control médico periódico.* —Patient in stable general condition, with vital signs within normal limits. She presents for follow-up of a chronic condition, reporting no new symptoms or warning signs. Denies fever, pain, shortness of breath, or other relevant clinical manifestations. On examination, she appears in good general condition, alert, oriented, and with adequate nutritional and hydration status. Physical exam is within normal parameters, with no evidence of localized or systemic compromise. Current management is maintained without changes, and periodic medical follow-up is advised.

These summaries clearly communicate that the patient is stable and that no urgent medical issues were identified during the exam. They avoid subjective language and provide a professional overview appropriate for the medical record.

**3  Tips for Writing Clear and Accurate Reports**

- ◉ Use neutral, descriptive language.
- ◉ Avoid assumptions or diagnostic conclusions unless supported by objective findings.
- ◉ Be brief but thorough —include relevant details without excessive commentary.
- ◉ Write in complete, grammatically correct Spanish using accepted medical terminology.
- ◉ Ensure that summaries are free from ambiguity and understandable to other clinicians.

Concise and accurate clinical reports are vital tools for documentation, collaboration, and patient safety. Writing clearly in Spanish enhances the accessibility and usability of medical records in bilingual or Spanish-speaking healthcare settings.

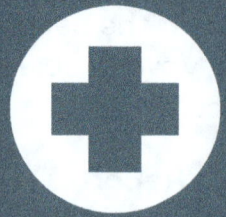

BOOK 4

# DISCUSSING DIAGNOSIS AND TREATMENT WITH SPANISH-SPEAKING PATIENTS

## A MEDICAL PROFESSIONAL'S GUIDE TO EXPLAINING TESTS, RESULTS, AND HEALTHCARE OPTIONS

ACQUIRE A LOT

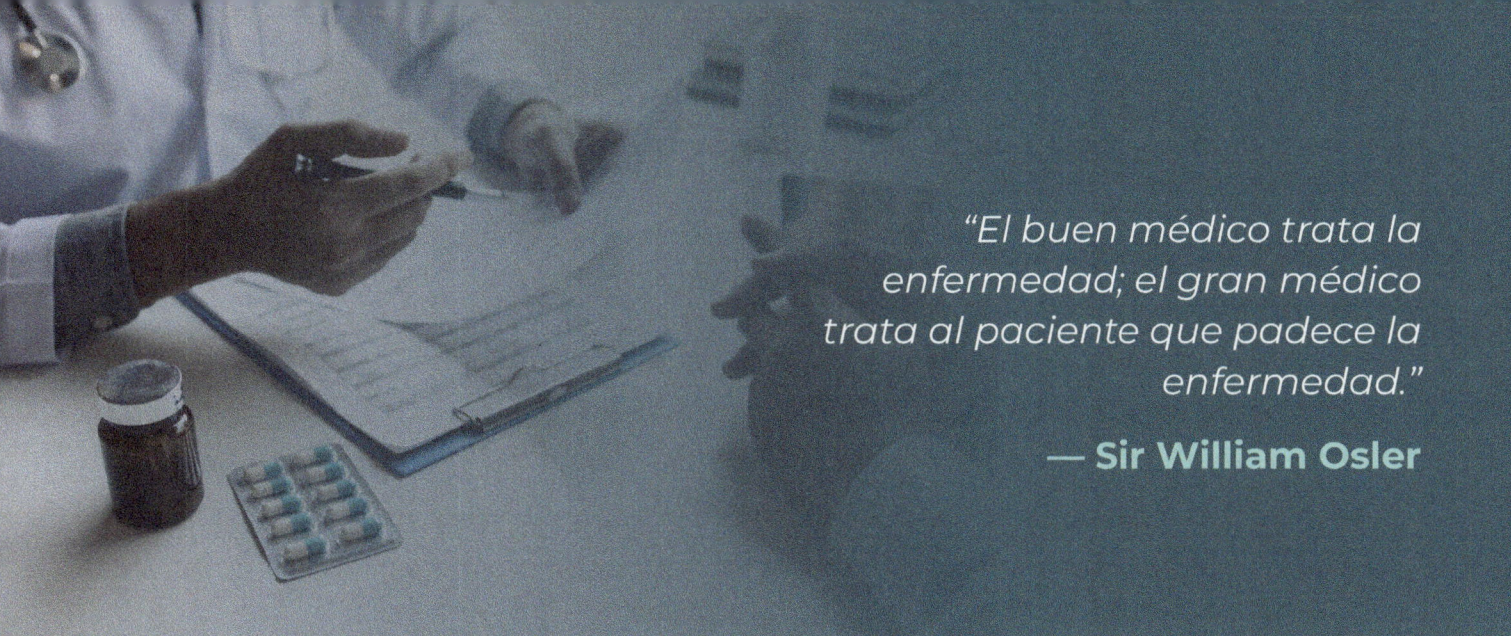

*"El buen médico trata la enfermedad; el gran médico trata al paciente que padece la enfermedad."*

— **Sir William Osler**

## CHAPTER 7

# EXPLAINING DIAGNOSTIC TESTS TO PATIENTS

## 7.1 Introducing the Need for Diagnostic Tests

Introducing diagnostic tests in a clear, respectful, and non-threatening manner is a vital skill in clinical practice. For many patients, especially those facing language or cultural barriers, the prospect of undergoing medical testing can provoke uncertainty or anxiety. How we explain the test affects how comfortable patients feel and if they follow through.

In Spanish-speaking clinical encounters, offering a thoughtful and transparent explanation in the patient's preferred language builds trust and promotes informed participation. Patients who understand why a test is necessary and how it contributes to their care are more likely to engage in follow-up, ask questions, and feel empowered in their health journey.

### 1 The Importance of Explaining Diagnostic Tests

Diagnostic tests provide essential information for confirming or ruling out medical conditions, guiding treatment plans, and monitoring disease progression. Introducing these tests clearly and compassionately is part of holistic, patient-centered care.

### 2 Phrases to Use When Introducing Diagnostic Tests

Use the following Spanish phrases to introduce the concept of diagnostic testing in a calm and reassuring manner:

- *Vamos a hacer algunas pruebas para entender mejor su condición.* — We're going to run some tests to better understand your condition.

- *Estas pruebas nos ayudarán a encontrar la causa de sus síntomas.* — These tests will help us find the cause of your symptoms.
- *No se preocupe, le explicaré cada paso.* — Don't worry, I'll explain each step.

**3  Best Practices When Discussing Tests**

- Use clear, non-technical language that the patient can understand.
- Emphasize the value of the test in helping to identify or rule out possible causes of symptoms.
- Acknowledge any concerns the patient may have, and offer space for questions.
- Reassure the patient that you will guide them through the process.
- If applicable, explain the next steps after the test is completed (e.g., when results will be ready, possible outcomes).

Diagnostic testing is a fundamental component of modern medicine. By taking the time to explain its purpose and process in Spanish, healthcare professionals help patients feel more informed, respected, and confident. This approach not only improves patient satisfaction but also enhances adherence to diagnostic and treatment plans, ultimately supporting better clinical outcomes.

## 7.2 Describing Common Laboratory Tests (Blood Test, Urine Analysis)

Laboratory tests are routine yet essential tools in the diagnostic process. They allow healthcare providers to assess organ function, detect infections, evaluate chronic disease markers, and monitor treatment effectiveness. For patients, however, these tests can be a source of confusion or concern—especially if instructions are not clearly communicated or if the purpose of the test is not fully explained.

In Spanish-speaking healthcare encounters, explaining what the test is for and how to prepare helps patients feel calm and cooperate. When patients understand what to expect, they are more likely to participate actively in their care and return for follow-up as needed.

**1  Blood Work and Urine Analysis**

Blood and urine tests are among the most frequently ordered diagnostics. These tests can evaluate a wide range of conditions, from diabetes to kidney function to infection. Clear communication in Spanish ensures patients know what will happen, why it is important, and whether any preparation is required.

**2  Sample Phrases for Communicating with Patients**

Use the following Spanish phrases to clearly explain laboratory testing procedures:

- *Vamos a tomar una muestra de sangre.* — We're going to take a blood sample.
- *Esta prueba mide su nivel de azúcar en la sangre.* — This test measures your blood sugar level.

- *También necesitamos una muestra de orina.* — We also need a urine sample.
- *No necesita estar en ayunas para esta prueba.* — You don't need to fast for this test.
- *Debe tener un ayuno de al menos 8 horas para hacerse este examen.* — You need to fast for at least 8 hours before taking this test.

### 3 Explaining Preparation and Instructions

Proper preparation is essential for accurate lab results. Some tests require fasting, specific timing, or stopping medications in advance. Always provide clear instructions, and ensure patients understand the reasoning behind them. For tests that do not require special preparation, reassuring the patient can help alleviate concern.

### 4 Best Practices for Discussing Lab Tests

- Use plain language to describe the test's purpose.
- Clarify any preparation requirements in advance.
- Reassure the patient about the safety and routine nature of the procedure.
- Encourage questions and provide written instructions if possible.
- Inform the patient of when and how results will be shared.

Lab tests are a critical part of modern diagnostics. By taking the time to explain them clearly in Spanish, healthcare providers reduce confusion, improve compliance, and strengthen the patient-provider relationship. These simple but essential conversations contribute significantly to high-quality, culturally competent care.

## 7.3 Explaining Imaging Procedures (X-ray, Ultrasound, CT scan, MRI)

Imaging procedures such as X-rays, ultrasounds, CT scans, and MRIs are invaluable tools in modern diagnostics. They allow clinicians to visualize structures inside the body with precision and are commonly used to detect fractures, organ abnormalities, tumors, and internal injuries. For many patients, especially those unfamiliar with medical imaging, the process can be intimidating or confusing.

Explaining in simple Spanish what to expect eases nerves and helps cooperation. It is especially important to mention whether the test involves radiation, produces noise, or requires stillness or special positioning.

### 1 Why Imaging Tests Are Important

Imaging tests help providers evaluate structures that cannot be assessed through physical examination alone. They are crucial for diagnosing internal conditions and planning treatment. When patients understand the purpose of the test, they are more likely to feel comfortable and informed.

### 2 Helpful Spanish Phrases for Common Imaging Tests

Use the following Spanish phrases to introduce and explain imaging procedures:

- *Vamos a hacer una radiografía para ver sus huesos/pulmones.* — We're going to take an X-ray to see your bones/lungs.

- *El ultrasonido utiliza ondas sonoras, no radiación.* — Ultrasound uses sound waves, not radiation.

- *La tomografía computarizada toma imágenes detalladas del interior del cuerpo.* — The CT scan takes detailed images of the inside of the body.

- *La resonancia magnética puede hacer ruido, pero no causa dolor.* — The MRI may be noisy, but it is not painful.

- *Si siente incomodidad durante la resonancia magnética, avise de forma inmediata.* — If you feel any discomfort during the MRI, notify us immediately.

### 3 Addressing Patient Concerns About Imaging

Many patients may feel nervous about imaging due to fear of radiation, discomfort, or claustrophobia. Proactively addressing these concerns can enhance comfort and compliance. Clarify which tests involve radiation and explain that procedures like MRI or ultrasound are non-invasive and safe.

For instance, some common phrases include:

- *Quiero explicarle lo que vamos a hacer para que se sienta más tranquilo(a). Si tiene alguna duda o algo le incomoda, por favor dígamelo. Esto puede ayudar a que el procedimiento sea más cómodo para usted.* — I'd like to explain what we're going to do so you can feel more at ease. If you have any questions or feel any discomfort, please let me know. This will help make the procedure more comfortable for you.

- *La ecografía es un examen indoloro, pero puede sentir un poco de presión cuando deslicemos el transductor sobre la piel. Si en algún momento siente molestia, por favor avise.* — The ultrasound is a painless exam, but you may feel some pressure as we move the transducer over your skin. If you feel any discomfort at any point, please let us know.

### 4 Best Practices When Discussing Imaging

- Always explain what the test is and what it is used for.
- Reassure the patient that most imaging tests are quick and painless.
- Mention if they need to lie still, remove metal objects, or follow other special instructions.
- Encourage questions and provide follow-up information about when results will be available.

Explaining imaging procedures clearly in Spanish helps patients feel informed, safe, and respected. By addressing both the purpose and the experience of the test, providers strengthen trust and promote a smoother diagnostic process. Patient-centered communication is a key component of high-quality, culturally competent care.

## 7.4 Describing Endoscopic Procedures (Colonoscopy, Gastroscopy)

Endoscopic procedures such as colonoscopy and gastroscopy are important diagnostic tools that allow direct visualization of internal structures. These minimally invasive techniques are used to examine the gastrointestinal tract, detect abnormalities, collect tissue samples, and even perform therapeutic interventions. For many patients, the idea of undergoing an endoscopy can cause anxiety. Clear, professional communication, especially in the patient's preferred language, is essential to prepare them emotionally and physically.

### 1  The Role of Endoscopic Procedures in Diagnosis

Colonoscopy and gastroscopy provide valuable insight into the health of the gastrointestinal tract. These procedures are often recommended to investigate symptoms such as abdominal pain, bleeding, or digestive issues. They are also important for cancer screening and follow-up.

### 2  Helpful Spanish Phrases to Describe the Procedures

Use these Spanish phrases to explain endoscopic procedures in a clear and calming manner:

- *Una colonoscopia examina el intestino grueso usando una cámara.* — A colonoscopy examines the large intestine using a camera.
- *La gastroscopia permite observar el esófago, el estómago y el duodeno.* — Gastroscopy allows visualization of the esophagus, stomach, and duodenum.
- *Estará sedado(a) durante el procedimiento para que no sienta molestias.* — You'll be sedated during the procedure so you won't feel discomfort.
- *Es posible que se deban obtener algunas muestras de tejidos o biopsias durante su examen, pero las molestias serán mínimas* — It may be necessary to take some tissue samples or biopsies during your exam, but any discomfort will be minimal.

### 3  Preparing the Patient for the Procedure

Preparation is essential for successful outcomes. Patients should be informed of dietary restrictions, the use of laxatives (in the case of colonoscopy), and the need for a responsible adult to accompany them if sedation is used. Explaining the sedation process helps relieve fear and promotes cooperation.

In Spanish, you could say:

- *Deberá realizar una preparación para su colonoscopia, que consiste en una dieta especial y la toma de un laxante* — You will need to follow a preparation for your colonoscopy, which includes a special diet and taking a laxative.
- *Su examen de colonoscopia/gastroscopia será realizado bajo una sedación suave* — Your colonoscopy/gastroscopy will be performed under mild sedation.
- *Para realizar la gastroscopia debe realizar un ayuno de mínimo 6 horas* — You must fast for at least 6 hours before the gastroscopy.

Patients should also be encouraged to ask questions and share any previous experiences or medical conditions that may affect sedation or tolerance.

**4** **Best Practices for Explaining Endoscopy**

- Use simple, reassuring language when describing the procedure and preparation.
- Emphasize the importance of following preparation instructions for safety and accuracy.
- Clarify that sedation will keep the patient comfortable and minimize awareness during the test.
- Encourage patients to express concerns or ask about aftercare and recovery.

Endoscopic procedures can be highly effective and insignificant risk when patients are well-informed and properly prepared. Providing this information in Spanish promotes understanding, reduces anxiety, and helps ensure the procedure goes smoothly. Clear communication is central to delivering respectful, safe, and culturally competent care.

## 7.5 Explaining Cardiac Tests (ECG, Echocardiogram)

Cardiac diagnostic tests such as the electrocardiogram (ECG) and echocardiogram are crucial for evaluating heart health. They provide detailed insights into cardiac rhythm, structure, and function—helping clinicians detect arrhythmia, structural abnormalities, and heart disease. Because the heart is often associated with serious health concerns, patients may experience anxiety when these tests are recommended.

In Spanish-speaking settings, clearly explaining the purpose, process, and comfort level of cardiac tests is essential for building trust and encouraging compliance. Using straightforward and reassuring language helps reduce fear and improves the overall patient experience.

**1** **Why Cardiac Tests Matter**

Cardiac tests are commonly used to investigate symptoms such as chest pain, shortness of breath, dizziness, or palpitations. They are also used in routine checkups for patients with risk factors like high blood pressure, diabetes, or a family history of heart disease. When explained effectively, these tests become less intimidating and more empowering for the patient.

**2** **Helpful Spanish Phrases for Explaining Cardiac Tests**

Use these Spanish phrases to describe the procedures clearly and reassure the patient:

- *El electrocardiograma registra la actividad eléctrica del corazón.* — The ECG records the electrical activity of the heart.
- *El electrocardiograma es un procedimiento rápido e indoloro.* — The EKG is a quick and painless procedure.
- *El ecocardiograma usa ultrasonido, ondas sonoras, para ver cómo late su corazón.* — An echocardiogram uses sound waves (ultrasound) to show how your heart beats.

### 3  Preparing the Patient and Setting Expectations

While no extensive preparation is usually needed for these tests, it's helpful to inform patients that:

- *Para el electrocardiograma se le colocarán unos electrodos en la piel de su pecho, brazos y piernas. No es un procedimiento doloroso* — For an ECG, electrodes will be placed on the chest, arms, and legs.

- *El examen toma solo unos pocos minutos y no es doloroso. Por favor, permanezca lo más quieto posible.* — The test takes only a few minutes and does not cause pain. Please remain as still as possible.

- *Para realizar el ecocardiograma se le aplicará un gel en su pecho que se siente frío y se empleará un transductor para capturar las imágenes* — For an echocardiogram, gel will be applied to your chest — it may feel cold — and a transducer will be used to capture ultrasound images.

- *Los pacientes deben informar cualquier síntoma que presenten* — Patients should report any symptoms they're experiencing.

### 4  Best Practices for Cardiac Test Discussions

- Use calm, empathetic language when introducing tests.
- Emphasize the non-invasive and safe nature of the procedures.
- Allow time for questions and encourage the patient to express concerns.
- Provide information on when and how results will be shared.

Cardiac tests are essential to diagnosing and managing heart conditions, but they can be intimidating if not properly explained. By using clear and compassionate communication in Spanish, healthcare providers can ease fears, build trust, and ensure patients are engaged and informed participants in their cardiac care.

### Caso Clínico

*Este ejercicio integra diversos conceptos que van desde la evaluación clínica hasta las opciones de tratamiento, y busca promover la reflexión sobre la importancia de la integración clínica, la toma de decisiones oportuna y la comunicación efectiva con el paciente en escenarios cardiovasculares de alto riesgo. El caso se presenta de manera bilingüe (español-inglés) con el fin de apoyar simultáneamente el aprendizaje del idioma y el razonamiento clínico, permitiendo a los profesionales de la salud fortalecer tanto sus habilidades en español médico como sus capacidades diagnósticas.*

### Clinical Case

This exercise integrates various concepts ranging from clinical assessment to treatment options, encouraging reflection on the importance of clinical integration, timely decision-making, and effective patient communication in high-risk cardiovascular scenarios. The case is presented bilingually (Spanish-English) to support language learning and clinical reasoning simultaneously, allowing healthcare professionals to strengthen both their medical Spanish skills and diagnostic abilities.

### Historia Clínica

*La señora López es una mujer de 60 años que acude a la consulta médica con síntomas de dolor en el pecho y dificultad para respirar durante las últimas 48 horas. Ha tenido antecedentes de hipertensión y diabetes tipo 2.*

### Clinical History

Ms. López is a 60-year-old woman who presents to the medical consultation with symptoms of chest pain and shortness of breath over the past 48 hours. She has a medical history of high blood pressure and type 2 diabetes.

### Hallazgos de la exploración física

- *Frecuencia cardíaca: 100 latidos por minuto.*
- *Presión arterial: 160/100 mmHg.*
- *Frecuencia respiratoria: 22 respiraciones por minuto.*
- *Auscultación pulmonar: Se escuchan crepitaciones en las bases de ambos pulmones.*

### Physical Examination Findings

The patient has a heart rate of 100 beats per minute and a blood pressure of 160/100 mmHg. Her respiratory rate is 22 breaths per minute. Pulmonary auscultation reveals crackles at the bases of both lungs.

### Pruebas diagnósticas:

- *Electrocardiograma (ECG): Presencia de ondas Q en derivaciones DII, DIII y aVF, con inversión persistente de la onda T.*
- *Análisis de sangre: Elevación leve de troponinas cardíacas: Troponina I (cTnI): 0,14 ng/mL y Troponina T (cTnT): 0,05 ng/mL. Péptido natriurético cerebral (BNP): 1450 pg/mL.*
- *Radiografía de tórax: Evidencia signos de congestión pulmonar y sobrecarga de volumen.*

### Diagnostic Test

The electrocardiogram (ECG) shows the presence of Q waves in leads II, III, and aVF, along with persistent T-wave inversion, suggesting a prior inferior myocardial infarction. Blood tests reveal mildly elevated cardiac troponin levels: Troponin I (cTnI) at 0.14 ng/mL and Troponin T (cTnT) at 0.05 ng/mL. The B-type natriuretic peptide (BNP) level is significantly elevated at 1450 pg/mL, indicating possible heart failure. The chest X-ray demonstrates signs of pulmonary congestion and volume overload.

### Impresión diagnóstica

*Basándose en los síntomas, los hallazgos de la exploración física y los resultados de las pruebas diagnósticas, el médico sospecha que la señora López ha sufrido un infarto de miocardio (ataque al corazón) que la está llevando a una insuficiencia cardíaca congestiva asociada.*

### Diagnostic Impression

Based on the symptoms, physical examination findings, and diagnostic test results, the physician suspects that Ms. López has suffered a myocardial infarction (heart attack), which has led to associated congestive heart failure.

### Explicación al paciente

*Médico: "Señora López, después de evaluar sus síntomas y realizar algunas pruebas, creemos que puede haber sufrido un ataque al corazón. Esto significa que una parte de su corazón no ha recibido suficiente sangre debido a una obstrucción en una de las arterias coronarias. Además, hemos notado signos de congestión en sus pulmones, lo que sugiere que su corazón no está bombeando tan eficientemente como debería."*

*Paciente: "¿Qué significa esto para mí? ¿Qué tratamiento necesito?"*

*Médico: "Vamos a iniciar un tratamiento para ayudar a su corazón a recuperarse y prevenir futuros problemas. Esto puede incluir medicamentos para evitar la formación de coágulos en su sangre, reducir la presión arterial y mejorar la función cardíaca. También es posible que necesitemos realizar una angiografía coronaria para ver exactamente dónde está la obstrucción y decidir si necesitamos realizar una intervención para recanalizar la arteria afectada."*

*Paciente: "¿Y qué puedo hacer para prevenir que esto vuelva a suceder?"*

*Médico: "Hay varias cosas que puede hacer para mejorar su salud cardíaca. Esto incluye seguir una dieta saludable baja en grasas saturadas y sal, realizar ejercicio regularmente, dejar de fumar si lo hace, y procurar que quienes conviven con usted también eviten fumar, y tomar sus medicamentos según lo prescrito. También es importante controlar su presión arterial y niveles de azúcar en sangre."*

### Explanation to the patient:

Doctor: "Mrs. López, after evaluating your symptoms and performing some tests, we believe you may have had a heart attack. This means that part of your heart has not received enough blood due to a blockage in one of the coronary arteries. In addition, we have noticed signs of congestion in your lungs, which suggests that your heart is not pumping as efficiently as it should."

Patient: "What does this mean for me? What treatment do I need?"

Doctor: "We're going to start a treatment plan to help your heart recover and prevent future problems. This may include medications to prevent blood clots, lower your blood pressure, and improve heart function. We may also need to perform a coronary angiography to see exactly where the blockage is and decide whether an intervention is needed to reopen the affected artery."

Patient: "And what can I do to prevent this from happening again?"

Doctor: "There are several things you can do to improve your heart health. These include following a healthy diet low in saturated fats and salt, exercising regularly, quitting smoking if you smoke — and encouraging those who live with you to avoid smoking as well — and taking your medications as prescribed. It's also important to keep your blood pressure and blood sugar levels under control."

### *Plan de tratamiento*

- *Ingreso hospitalario para monitoreo y tratamiento intensivo en Unidad de Cuidados Coronarios.*
- *Administración de medicamentos para el infarto de miocardio y la insuficiencia cardíaca.*
- *Evaluación por cardiología para considerar angiografía coronaria y posible intervención.*
- *Educación al paciente sobre cambios en el estilo de vida y manejo de enfermedades crónicas.*

### Treatment Plan

- The patient will be admitted to the Coronary Care Unit (CCU) for close monitoring and intensive treatment.
- Medications will be administered to address both the myocardial infarction and the associated heart failure.
- A cardiology evaluation will be conducted to assess the need for a coronary angiography and determine whether an interventional procedure is required.
- Additionally, the patient will receive education focused on lifestyle changes and the long-term management of chronic conditions.

### *Análisis*

*Este caso clínico ilustra la importancia de comunicar de manera clara y compasiva la hipótesis diagnóstica y el plan de tratamiento a los pacientes, asegurándose de que comprendan su condición y los pasos necesarios para su recuperación y manejo a largo plazo.*

### Analysis

This clinical case illustrates the importance of clearly and compassionately communicating the diagnostic impression and treatment plan to patients, ensuring they understand their condition and the steps necessary for their recovery and long-term management.

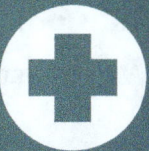

CHAPTER 8

# DISCUSSING TEST RESULTS AND DIAGNOSES

## 8.1 Explaining Normal and Abnormal Test Results Clearly

Sharing test results is one of the most important moments in the patient-provider relationship. Whether the findings are normal or abnormal, the way in which results are communicated significantly affects patient understanding, emotional response, and trust in the care process. Clarity, empathy, and cultural sensitivity are essential—especially in Spanish-speaking clinical settings.

When explaining results, providers should use plain language, avoid medical jargon, and offer reassurance while still being honest. Encouraging patients to ask questions and involving them in next steps helps build confidence and promotes shared decision-making.

### 1 Communicating Normal Results

It is important to share good news clearly and confidently. Even when test results are within normal limits, patients benefit from understanding what that means in the context of their symptoms or concerns.

Useful expressions when communicating normal results to the patient:

- *Sus resultados están dentro de un rango normal / Sus resultados son normales.* — Your results are within the normal range / Your results are normal.

- This statement can be followed by a brief explanation of the tested parameters and reassurance that no signs of concern were found. This also provides an opportunity to educate the patient about warning signs relevant to their condition. For example:

- *Su nivel de glucemia en ayunas no debe superar 100 mg/dL.* — Your fasting blood glucose level should not exceed 100 mg/dL.

- *Su presión arterial debe mantenerse por debajo de 120/80 mmHg.* — Your blood pressure should stay below 120/80 mmHg.

### ② Communicating Abnormal Findings with Care

When test results reveal abnormalities, communication should be clear, calm, and supportive. Patients need to understand what was found, what it might mean, and what the next steps will be. Avoid overwhelming them with complex details; instead, present information in manageable, compassionate language.

Appropriate wording:

- *Hemos encontrado algo anormal en los resultados, debemos investigar más las posibles causas.* — We found something abnormal in the results and need to investigate further to determine the possible causes.

Then explain whether the finding is urgent, what possible causes are being considered, and the next steps in the evaluation. This helps the patient understand the next steps and reduces uncertainty or anxiety about the findings.

### ③ When Additional Testing is Needed

Sometimes results are inconclusive or suggest the need for further evaluation. Reassuring the patient that more testing is a common and precautionary step can help reduce anxiety.

Model phrases you can use:

- *Necesitamos hacer más estudios para confirmar el diagnóstico.* — We need to do more tests to confirm the diagnosis.

Be sure to explain what types of tests are being recommended, the timeframe in which they should be performed, and what you are looking to evaluate. Patients should feel well-informed and empoweredto actively participate in their care plan.

Phrases Commonly Used:

- *El ideal es realizar una ecocardiografía antes de los próximos tres días para evaluar cómo está funcionando su corazón. Esta prueba nos permitirá identificar si hay algún problema con la fuerza de contracción o con las válvulas. Es importante que asista puntualmente, ya que esta información nos ayudará a decidir el tratamiento más adecuado para usted.* — Ideally, an echocardiogram should be performed within the next three days to evaluate how your heart is functioning. This test will help us identify any issues with the heart's pumping strength or the valves. It is important that you attend the appointment on time, as this information will help us determine the most appropriate treatment for you.

### ④ Best Practices for Discussing Test Results

Here are some best practices to ensure effective communication:

- Use calm, non-technical language.
- Give patients space to process the information.
- Encourage questions and invite participation in decisions.

- Provide written summaries when appropriate.
- Follow up to ensure understanding and continuity of care.

How test results are communicated can shape a patient's entire healthcare experience. By explaining findings clearly in Spanish, providers demonstrate respect, professionalism, and empathy—essential qualities in effective, culturally responsive care.

## 8.2 Communicating a Diagnosis with Sensitivity and Clarity

Communicating a diagnosis can have a profound impact on the clinician-patient relationship. Whether the diagnosis is routine or life-altering, the provider's ability to speak with compassion, clarity, and cultural awareness profoundly shapes the patient's experience. This is especially true when working with Spanish-speaking patients who may have added barriers to understanding due to language or unfamiliarity with the healthcare system.

Effective communication during this time helps reduce fear, increase comprehension, and empowers patients to take part actively in managing their health. It also lays the groundwork for trust and long-term engagement in care.

### 1 Approaching the Diagnosis Conversation

When delivering a diagnosis, the tone and language used are just as important as the information itself. Start by confirming that the patient is ready to hear the results, then go ahead at a pace that allows for emotional and cognitive processing.

One common way to say it is:

- *Afortunadamente, los resultados indican que no hay signos de...* — Fortunately, the results indicate there are no signs of...
- *Lamentablemente, los resultados indican que tiene...* — Unfortunately, the results indicate you have...

Use this phrase gently, followed by a clear explanation of the condition, its implications, and the next steps.

The following sample statements illustrate the recommended approach:

- *Usted tiene una condición llamada [nombre de la enfermedad]. Esto significa que...* — You have a condition called [name of condition]. This means...
- *Esta enfermedad afecta a [órgano o sistema], y puede causar [síntomas]....* — This condition affects the [organ or system] and can cause [symptoms]...
- *Vamos a trabajar juntos para manejar esta condición de la mejor manera posible.* — We'll work together to manage this condition as best as possible.

- *Entiendo que esto puede ser difícil de oír, pero estoy aquí para acompañarle y explicarle todo con calma.* — I understand this may be difficult to hear, but I'm here to support you and explain everything clearly.

### 2  Explaining Diagnoses Clearly and Compassionately

Clearly and compassionately explaining a diagnosis is a vital healthcare skill. It helps patients understand their condition, fosters trust, and supports shared decision-making. Spanish-speaking patients often face language barriers that can prevent them from fully grasping complex medical explanations. This section equips healthcare professionals with strategies and phrases to explain diagnoses effectively in Spanish, using a tone that is both professional and empathetic.

Phrasing options:

- *Lo que usted tiene se llama [nombre de la enfermedad/condición]. Significa que...* — What you have is called [name of the disease/condition]. It means that...

- *Sé que esta información puede ser difícil de recibir y entender. Estoy aquí para explicarle lo que necesite y listo a responder sus preguntas.* — I know this information may be difficult to receive and understand. I'm here to explain anything you need and ready to answer your questions.

### 3  Offering Treatment Options and Support

Patients often feel overwhelmed when they hear a diagnosis, especially if it is unexpected or serious. Offering treatment options or reassurance that the condition is manageable can provide comfort and restore a sense of control.

In Spanish, you could say:

- *Esta condición se puede tratar/controlar con...* — This condition can be treated/managed with...

When possible, share success stories, outline the treatment plan, and explain what support will be available.

### 4  Being Present and Available for the Patient

Communicating a diagnosis is not a one-time task. It is a process that may involve multiple conversations. Reassure  the patient that they are not alone, and that you are committed to walking with them through their care journey.

For instance, some common phrases include:

- *Estoy aquí para ayudarle a entender y a manejar esto.* — I'm here to help you understand and manage this.

*Puede contar con mi apoyo y el de todo el equipo que lo va a atender para manejar esto.* — You can count on my support and on the entire care team to help you manage this

**⑤ Best Practices for Communicating Diagnoses**

- ⊙ Ensure privacy and a quiet setting.
- ⊙ Avoid rushing—allow time for emotions and questions.
- ⊙ Speak slowly and use plain language.
- ⊙ Check for understanding and emotional response.
- ⊙ Offer written materials or resources when right.

Delivering a diagnosis is a deep human interaction that requires emotional intelligence as well as clinical knowledge. By approaching the conversation with empathy and linguistic clarity, especially in Spanish-speaking encounters, providers can help patients feel supported and equipped to face the path ahead. These conversations are not just about delivering news—they are opportunities to prove care.

## 8.3 Discussing Differential Diagnoses

In many clinical scenarios, a definitive diagnosis may not be possible at once. Instead, providers must consider a range of possible explanations for a patient's symptoms. This is known as the differential diagnosis. Effectively communicating this uncertainty requires transparency, reassurance, and collaboration. Spanish-speaking patients, in particular, should be informed that further testing and time may be necessary before a final diagnosis is confirmed.

When managed well, these discussions build trust and help patients understand that clinical decision-making is a thoughtful and thorough process. By using understandable language and encouraging patient engagement, providers can foster a supportive and respectful diagnostic experience.

**① Explaining the Need for a Differential Diagnosis**

Introducing the concept of differential diagnosis helps the patient understand that medicine often involves ruling out several possibilities before arriving at a definitive answer. Providers should explain this process with patience and clarity.

Possible phrasing:

- ⊙ *Podría ser una de varias condiciones...* — It could be one of several conditions...
- ⊙ *En este momento, hay varias posibles causas para sus síntomas. Vamos a hacer algunas pruebas para entender mejor qué está ocurriendo y asegurarnos de darle el tratamiento correcto.* —Right now, there are several possible causes for your symptoms. We're going to run some tests to better understand what's going on and make sure you receive the right treatment.

## 2  Communicating the Plan for Further Evaluation

When a diagnosis is uncertain, outlining the next steps can reassure the patient and clarify the path forward. This might include laboratory testing, imaging, specialist referrals, or follow-up appointments. Being transparent about the process helps reduce anxiety.

Possible phrasing:

⊙ *Vamos a hacer más pruebas para confirmar el diagnóstico.* — We'll do more tests to confirm the diagnosis.

## 3  Describing the Purpose of Testing

It is important to help patients understand that not all tests are designed to confirm a specific diagnosis and many are used to rule out other conditions. This initiative-taking approach shows that the provider is being thorough and careful in their evaluation.

Possible phrasing:

⊙ *Esto nos ayudará a descartar otras posibilidades.* — This will help us rule out other possibilities.

## 4  Best Practices for Managing Diagnostic Uncertainty

⊙ Be honest and open about diagnostic uncertainty.

⊙ Avoid overwhelming the patient with medical terminology.

⊙ Offer a clear and actionable plan.

⊙ Emphasize that exploring multiple possibilities is a hallmark of thorough medical care.

⊙ Encourage the patient to stay engaged and to follow up as recommended.

Differential diagnosis is a fundamental part of clinical reasoning. While uncertainty can be challenging, it also presents an opportunity to build trust through clear and thoughtful communication. For Spanish-speaking patients, explaining the process respectfully and in their preferred language helps them feel informed, supported, and empowered throughout their healthcare journey.

## 8.4 Addressing Patient Questions and Concerns About Test Results

Discussing test results can be a moment of anxiety for many patients. Whether the news is reassuring or concerning, patients often have questions, doubts, or emotional responses that need to be acknowledged. Effective communication in this context is not only about providing exact information, but also about being present, empathetic, and responsive.

For Spanish-speaking patients, this process must also be linguistically and culturally appropriate. Healthcare providers should create space for questions, explain results in understandable language, and offer reassurance when possible. These conversations build patient confidence, strengthen the therapeutic relationship, and ensure informed decision-making.

### 1 Inviting the Patient to Ask Questions

Be sure to let patients know they are welcome to ask questions. This reduces uncertainty and encourages open dialogue. Providers should pause after sharing the results, giving the patient time to reflect and ask questions.

Example Phrase:

- *Quiero asegurarme de que todo haya quedado claro. ¿Tiene alguna duda sobre los resultados?* — I want to make sure everything is clear. Do you have any questions about the results?

### 2 Showing Empathy and Understanding

Receiving medical results can be emotionally complex. Providers should acknowledge this and respond in a calm, supportive tone. This helps patients feel seen and heard, even when outcomes are uncertain or difficult.

Sample questions for gathering information:

- *Entiendo que esto puede ser confuso.* — I understand this may be confusing.
- *Entiendo que pueda estar confundido(a).* — I understand you may be feeling confused.

### 3 Walking Through the Results Collaboratively

Many patients benefit from a step-by-step review of their results. By explaining each section of a report and pausing questions, providers can make technical information accessible and meaningful.

Example Phrase:

- *Podemos revisar los resultados juntos, paso a paso.* — We can review the results together, step by step.

### 4 Best Practices for Managing Patient Concerns

- Use visual aids or written materials when appropriate.
- Speak slowly and avoid medical jargon.
- Allow time for silence and processing.
- Encourage follow-up conversations if needed.
- Always reassure the patient that their concerns are valid and valued.

Creating a space where patients feel comfortable asking questions and expressing concerns is a hallmark of care that feels respectful and kind. When providers communicate results with empathy and clarity—especially in Spanish-language interactions—they help patients feel more informed, less anxious, and more engaged in their care.

### Caso Clínico

*Este caso clínico destaca la importancia de discutir los resultados de las pruebas y el diagnóstico con el paciente de manera clara y comprensiva, asegurándose de que comprenda su enfermedad y el plan de tratamiento propuesto.*

*El paciente es el señor Martínez, un hombre de 45 años que acude a consulta médica por dolor abdominal y diarrea crónica de varios meses de evolución. En su historia clínica se documenta que el señor Martínez ha estado experimentando dolor abdominal y diarrea durante los últimos 6 meses, ha presentado pérdida de peso progresiva y ha notado sangre en sus heces en varias ocasiones.*

### Clinical Case

This clinical case highlights the importance of discussing test results and diagnosis with the patient in a clear and compassionate manner, ensuring they understand their condition and the proposed treatment plan.

The patient is Mr. Martínez, a 45-year-old man who comes to the clinic due to abdominal pain and chronic diarrhea of several months' duration. His medical history reveals he has been experiencing abdominal pain and diarrhea for the past six months, with progressive weight loss and occasional blood in his stools.

### Pruebas diagnósticas

- *Colonoscopia: Se observan lesiones ulceradas localizadas en colon sigmoide y recto, de las cuales se tomaron biopsias.*

- *Histopatología: Las biopsias revelan inflamación crónica de la mucosa con presencia de ulceraciones, hallazgos sugestivos de colitis ulcerosa.*

- *Análisis de laboratorio: Anemia leve, elevación de marcadores inflamatorios (PCR y VSG) y elevación de la Calprotectina fecal.*

### Diagnostic Tests

- Colonoscopy: Ulcerated lesions are observed in the sigmoid colon and rectum, from which biopsies were taken.

- Histopathology: The biopsies show chronic mucosal inflammation with ulcerations, findings consistent with ulcerative colitis.

- Laboratory analysis: Mild anemia, elevated inflammatory markers (CRP and ESR), and elevated fecal calprotectin.

### Discusión de resultados y diagnóstico

*Médico: "Señor Martínez, hemos recibido los resultados de las pruebas que le realizamos. La endoscopia mostró úlceras en su colon y recto, y la biopsia confirmó el diagnóstico de colitis ulcerosa. Esta es una enfermedad inflamatoria crónica del intestino que causa úlceras e inflamación en el revestimiento del colon y recto."*

Paciente: *"¿Qué significa esto para mí? ¿Cómo afectará mi vida diaria?"*

Médico: *"La colitis ulcerosa puede causar síntomas como diarrea con sangre, dolor abdominal y pérdida de peso. Aunque no tiene cura, hay tratamientos efectivos para controlar los síntomas y reducir la inflamación. Podemos hablar sobre opciones de tratamiento que incluyen medicamentos antiinflamatorios, inmunomoduladores y, en algunos casos, cirugía."*

Paciente: *"¿Qué tipo de cambios en mi estilo de vida necesito hacer?"*

Médico: *"Es importante llevar una dieta equilibrada y evitar alimentos que, en su caso particular, puedan agravar los síntomas, como los muy grasos, picantes o ricos en fibra insoluble. También es crucial tomar sus medicamentos según lo prescrito y asistir a citas de seguimiento regulares para monitorear su condición. Además, podemos discutir estrategias para manejar el estrés, que puede influir en su enfermedad."*

## Discussion of Results and Diagnosis

Doctor: "Mr. Martínez, we have received the results of the tests we performed. The endoscopy showed ulcers in your colon and rectum, and the biopsy confirmed the diagnosis of ulcerative colitis. This is a type of chronic inflammatory bowel disease that causes ulcers and inflammation in the lining of the colon and rectum."

Patient: "What does this mean for me? How will it affect my daily life?"

Doctor: "Ulcerative colitis can cause symptoms such as bloody diarrhea, abdominal pain, and weight loss. Although it has no cure, there are effective treatments to control symptoms and reduce inflammation. We can discuss treatment options including anti-inflammatory medications, immunosuppressants, and in some cases, surgery."

Patient: "What kind of lifestyle changes do I need to make?"

Doctor: "It is important to maintain a balanced diet and avoid foods that, in your particular case, may worsen your symptoms, such as very fatty, spicy foods, or those high in insoluble fiber. It is also crucial to take your medications as prescribed and attend regular follow-up appointments to monitor your condition. Additionally, we can discuss stress management strategies, as stress can influence your disease."

## *Plan de tratamiento*

- ⊙ *Medicamentos: Iniciar tratamiento con aminosalicilatos para reducir la inflamación y controlar los síntomas. Evaluar la necesidad de agregar corticosteroides en caso de Exacerbación moderada o severa del cuadro clínico.*
- ⊙ *Seguimiento: Citas regulares para monitorear la respuesta clínica y bioquímica al tratamiento iniciado, realizando los ajustes según la evolución y la tolerancia al mismo.*
- ⊙ *Educación: Brindar información clara sobre la enfermedad, los signos de alarma, el manejo de síntomas y las posibles complicaciones. Es clave analizar con el paciente los factores dietéticos protectores o agravantes de su alimentación actual.*

- *Apoyo: Referir al paciente a un grupo de apoyo para personas con enfermedades inflamatorias intestinales, con el fin de promover el acompañamiento emocional y el intercambio de experiencias.*

**Treatment Plan**

- Medications: Initiate treatment with aminosalicylates to reduce inflammation and control symptoms. Evaluate the need to add corticosteroids in case of moderate or severe exacerbation of the clinical picture.

- Follow-up: Regular appointments to monitor both clinical and biochemical response to treatment, making adjustments according to the evolution and tolerance.

- Education: Provide clear information about the disease, warning signs, symptom management, and possible complications. It is essential to discuss with the patient the protective or aggravating dietary factors in their current diet.

- Support: Refer the patient to a support group for individuals with inflammatory bowel disease to promote emotional support and sharing of experiences.

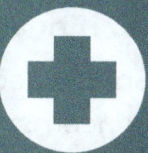

CHAPTER 9

# EXPLAINING TREATMENT OPTIONS

## 9.1 Introducing Different Treatment Modalities (Medication, Therapy, Surgery)

Explaining treatment options is a pivotal aspect of patient-centered care. It involves not only presenting the medically appropriate choices but also respecting the patient's values, concerns, and preferences. Especially in Spanish-speaking settings, the ability to communicate these options clearly and compassionately builds trust and encourages collaborative decision-making.

Every treatment—medicines, therapy, or surgery—has its pros and cons. We walk patients through their options in clear terms so they feel ready to choose.

**1  Outlining Available Treatments**

Begin by giving an overview of the possible treatment modalities, emphasizing that no decision needs to be made at once and that the patient will be supported throughout the process.

Language examples:

◉  *Existen diferentes opciones de tratamiento, incluyendo cirugía, medicamentos y apoyo psicológico.* — There are different treatment options, including surgery, medication, and psychological support.

**2  Explaining Pros and Cons of Each Option**

Clarify the purpose, benefits, and potential side effects of each option. Patients may have prior experiences or beliefs about treatments that influence their preferences. Respectful dialogue is key.

Language examples:

◉  *Le explicaré los beneficios y riesgos de cada opción.* — I will explain the benefits and risks of each option.

### 3   Engaging the Patient in the Decision Process

Shared decision-making reinforces the provider-patient partnership. Invite the patient to express concerns, ask questions, and reflect on how each treatment might affect their life.

Model phrases you can use:

- *Podemos decidir juntos cuál es el mejor plan para usted.* — We can decide together what the best plan is for you.

- *Podemos revisar sus opciones y elegir juntos la que se ajuste mejor a sus necesidades.* — We can go over your options and choose the one that best fits your needs together.

### 4   Best Practices for Presenting Treatment Options

- Use simple, jargon-free language.
- Check for understanding at each stage.
- Be honest about uncertainties or limitations.
- Encourage family involvement when appropriate.
- Offer printed materials in Spanish to support discussion.

Effectively introducing treatment options is not just a clinical task. It's a human connection. Spanish-speaking patients benefit most when providers explain clearly, listen attentively, and make space for shared choices. Empowering patients to make informed decisions creates stronger therapeutic alliances and improves overall care outcomes

## 9.2 Describing Medications: Dosage, Frequency, Route of Administration

Clear and accurate communication about medications is essential to ensure patient adherence, avoid errors, and maximize treatment outcomes. This is especially important when working with Spanish-speaking patients, where language barriers may increase the risk of misunderstanding instructions. Medication education must be adapted to the patient's level of health literacy, and all directions should be presented in an organized, respectful, and culturally sensitive way.

Healthcare providers must ensure that patients understand not only what medication to take, but also how much, how often, and by what route. Taking the time to explain these details in clear Spanish can prevent complications and increase a patient's confidence in their care plan.

### 1   Providing Dosage and Frequency Instructions

Patients need to know when and how often to take their medication. Clear explanations reduce the risk of over- or under-dosing.

Appropriate wording:

- *Debe tomar este medicamento así: una tableta una vez al día, por la mañana, al menos 30 minutos antes del desayuno.* — You should take this medication as follows: one tablet once a day, in the morning, at least 30 minutes before breakfast.

- *Debe tomar este medicamento así: una cucharada cada 8 horas, por ejemplo, a las 5 am, a las 1 pm y a las 10 pm, o en un horario similar.* — You should take this medication as follows: one tablespoon every 8 hours, for example at 5 a.m., 1 p.m., and 10 p.m., or at a similar schedule.

- *La dosis es de 500 miligramos cada 6 horas, por vía oral.* — The dose is 500 milligrams every 6 hours, taken orally.

### 2  Describing How the Medication is Taken

Some medications are taken by mouth, while others may be injected or given through an IV. Patients should clearly understand the route of administration to avoid errors and ensure proper use.

Appropriate wording:

- *El medicamento se administra por vía oral.* — The medication is administered orally.

- *Este medicamento puede administrarse mediante una inyección bajo la piel (subcutánea).* — This medication can be administered by injection under the skin (subcutaneously).

- *Este medicamento es para aplicación intravenosa (directamente en la vena).* — This medication is for intravenous administration (directly into the vein).

- *Su medicamento se administrará por vía intramuscular, en un músculo del glúteo o en el deltoides (ubicado en el hombro).* — Your medication will be administered intramuscularly, into a muscle in the buttock (gluteal) or the shoulder (deltoid).

### 3  Ensuring Patient Understanding

- Use visual aids or demonstrate when possible.

- Confirm understanding by asking the patient to repeat instructions in their own words.

- Provide written instructions in Spanish.

- Be patient and allow time for questions.

- Avoid complex medical terminology unless explained clearly.

Effectively describing medications in Spanish is a vital skill in clinical care. Precise instructions about dosage, timing, and route not only ensure medication safety but also empower patients to take control of their health. By communicating clearly and checking for understanding, healthcare professionals can significantly enhance treatment adherence and outcomes.

## 9.3 Explaining Surgical Procedures and Pre/Post-operative Instructions.

Explaining surgical procedures requires careful communication that balances technical accuracy with compassion and reassurance. For Spanish-speaking patients, understanding why a procedure is needed, what it involves, and how to prepare and recover is critical to informed consent, cooperation, and positive surgical outcomes.

Healthcare professionals must clearly outline the purpose of the surgery, any associated risks, and what the patient can expect before and after the operation. Providing this information in Spanish, and encouraging questions, ensures that patients feel supported and well-prepared.

### 1 Explaining the Purpose and Need for Surgery

Begin with a clear, direct explanation of why surgery is recommended and what benefit it will provide to the patient's condition.

Example Phrases:

- *Esta cirugía es necesaria para tratar su condición.* — This surgery is necessary to treat your condition.

- *Entendemos que es una decisión difícil, pero esta cirugía es necesaria para salvar su vida.* — We understand this is a difficult decision, but this surgery is necessary to save your life.

### 2 Giving Pre-operative Instructions

Patients need detailed guidance on how to prepare for surgery. This often includes fasting, medication restrictions, and logistical arrangements.

Sample expressions:

- *No debe comer ni beber nada la noche antes de la operación.* — You should not eat or drink the night before the surgery.

- *No debe comer ni beber nada 8 horas antes de la cirugía.* — You must not eat or drink anything for 8 hours before the surgery.

- *Por favor, llegue al hospital dos horas antes de la hora programada para la cirugía.* — Please arrive at the hospital two hours before your scheduled surgery time.

- *Debe retirarse desde la noche anterior todos los objetos personales como joyas, anillos, pulseras, maquillaje, esmalte de uñas y otros accesorios.* — You should remove all personal items the night before surgery, including jewelry, rings, bracelets, makeup, nail polish, and other accessories.

- *Debe suspender temporalmente algunos medicamentos antes de la operación; le indicaremos cuáles.* — You will need to temporarily stop taking certain medications before the operation; we will tell you which ones.

- *Necesitará que alguien lo acompañe y lo ayude una vez que salga de la sala de recuperación.* — You will need someone to accompany you and help you once you're out of the recovery room.

### 3 Outlining Post-operative Care and Recovery

Recovery requires patient cooperation with rest, wound care, medication, and follow-up appointments. Clear Spanish instructions help patients avoid complications and heal successfully.

Model phrases you can use:

- *Después de la cirugía, deberá descansar y seguir instrucciones específicas.* — After the surgery, you will need to rest and follow specific instructions.

- *Le daremos indicaciones claras sobre cómo tomar sus medicamentos y cuándo acudir a controles médicos.* — We will provide clear instructions on how to take your medications and when to attend follow-up appointments.

- *Asegúrese de mantener la zona de la cirugía limpia y seca, y evite esfuerzos físicos durante los próximos días.* — Ensure that you keep the surgical area clean and dry, and to avoid physical exertion for the next few days.

- *Si presenta fiebre, enrojecimiento, hinchazón excesiva o secreción en la zona de la cirugía, debe comunicarse con nosotros de inmediato.* — If you develop a fever, redness, excessive swelling, or discharge at the surgical site, you should contact us immediately.

### 4 Best Practices for Discussing Surgery

- Use visual aids or diagrams to explain the procedure.
- Provide written pre- and post-operative instructions in Spanish.
- Encourage patients to bring a family member to the discussion.
- Allow time for questions and clarify misconceptions.
- Be empathetic and validate concerns about surgery or recovery.

Discussing surgery with Spanish-speaking patients requires a thoughtful, structured approach that prioritizes understanding and emotional support. By explaining the purpose, process, and recovery steps clearly, providers empower patients to feel informed, prepared, and confident throughout their surgical journey.

## 9.4 Discussing Physical Therapy and Rehabilitation Plans

Physical therapy and rehabilitation are vital components of recovery for many patients. These therapies help restore movement, relieve pain, and improve physical function following surgery, injury, or chronic illness. For Spanish-speaking patients, it is essential to clearly explain the purpose, structure, and expectations of a physical therapy plan to ensure participation and maximize outcomes.

Healthcare professionals must communicate therapy goals, session schedules, and home exercises in an encouraging and culturally sensitive manner. Patients are more likely to commit to therapy when they understand its role in their recovery and how each step contributes to their progress.

### 1  Introducing the Need for Physical Therapy

Begin by clearly stating the reason for the therapy recommendation and how it will help with recovery or condition management.

In Spanish, you could do it this way:

- *Le recomendaremos fisioterapia para mejorar su movilidad.* — We will recommend physical therapy to improve your mobility.
- *Después de la cirugía, necesitará fisioterapia para recuperar la movilidad y fortalecer la zona afectada.* — After the surgery, you will need physical therapy to regain mobility and strengthen the affected area.

### 2  Outlining the Therapy Plan

Explain what the therapy plan will include—such as the types of exercises, frequency of sessions, and whether it will be supervised or done independently.

In Spanish, you could do it this way:

- *El plan incluirá ejercicios regulares y sesiones supervisadas.* — The plan will include regular exercises and supervised sessions.

### 3  Encouraging Participation and Consistency

Patient adherence is essential to the success of any rehabilitation plan. Stress the importance of showing up for all appointments and completing assigned exercises.

One common way to say it is

- *Es importante asistir a todas las sesiones para lograr buenos resultados.* — It's important to attend all sessions to achieve satisfactory results.

### 4  Best Practices for Therapy Communication

- Set clear and achievable therapy goals.
- Explain how progress will be measured.
- Provide written exercise instructions in Spanish.
- Encourage questions and address concerns about discomfort or fatigue.
- Reinforce the connection between therapy and long-term independence.

Discussing physical therapy with Spanish-speaking patients involves more than just outlining a plan—it requires motivation, support, and clarity. A well-explained rehabilitation plan helps patients regain confidence in their bodies and actively participate in their recovery. By ensuring clear communication and ongoing encouragement, providers can significantly improve patient outcomes.

## 9.5 Addressing Alternative and Complementary Therapies

In today's diverse healthcare landscape, many patients explore alternative and complementary therapies alongside conventional medical treatment. These may include acupuncture, herbal remedies, chiropractic care, homeopathy, or spiritual healing practices. For Spanish-speaking patients, it is important that providers create a welcoming environment for open dialogue about these interests.

When addressing alternative therapies, healthcare professionals should demonstrate respect for patients' beliefs and preferences, while also providing clear, evidence-informed guidance on safety and efficacy. This balanced approach fosters trust and helps patients make well-informed decisions about their care.

### 1 Recognizing the Use of Alternative Therapies

Acknowledging that many individuals may use or consider alternative therapies is the first step toward honest and transparent communication.

Model phrases you can use

- *Algunas personas usan tratamientos alternativos como acupuntura o hierbas.* — Some people use alternative treatments like acupuncture or herbs.

- *¿Cuáles tratamientos alternativos está utilizando actualmente?* — What alternative treatments are you currently using?

- *¿Puede decirme los nombres de los productos alternativos que está tomando?* — Can you tell me the names of the alternative products you are taking?

### 2 Providing a Balanced, Evidence-Informed Perspective

Encourage patients to discuss these therapies openly and be ready to provide information about known interactions or risks.

Model phrases you can use:

- *Si le interesa, podemos hablar sobre cuáles tratamientos alternativos son seguros y eficaces en algunos casos.* — If you're interested, we can talk about which alternative treatments are safe and effective in some cases.

### 3  Promoting Open Communication

Knowing about all therapies a patient is using helps healthcare providers avoid harmful interactions and provide truly holistic care.

Model phrases you can use

- ◉ *Siempre infórmenos si está usando otro tipo de terapia.* — Always let us know if you are using any other type of therapy.

- ◉ *Queremos que se sienta cómodo hablando con nosotros sobre cualquier tratamiento que esté realizando o cualquier duda que tenga.* — We want you to feel comfortable talking to us about any treatments you are using or any questions you may have.

### 4  Best Practices for These Conversations

- ◉ Listen respectfully and avoid dismissive language.
- ◉ Ask follow-up questions to understand the source and frequency of use.
- ◉ Document alternative therapy used in the patient's chart.
- ◉ Explain possible risks or interactions with current treatments.
- ◉ Support culturally sensitive dialogue with interpreters if needed.

Alternative and complementary therapies are increasingly common in modern healthcare. By addressing them with respect and clinical insight, providers can support informed decision-making, reinforce patient trust, and deliver safe, integrated healthcare. Encouraging honest dialogue ensures that all elements of a patient's care plan are known and considered.

### Caso Clínico

*Se recomienda desarrollar el ejercicio inicialmente en español, utilizando la versión en inglés como apoyo referencial. Aunque no se trata de una traducción literal, mantiene la equivalencia clínica y comunicativa, y puede servir como guía para estructurar la entrevista de manera clara y coherente.*

*Este caso clínico ilustra la importancia de explicar claramente las opciones de tratamiento al paciente, considerando sus necesidades individuales y preferencias, para asegurar una toma de decisiones informada y un manejo efectivo de la condición.*

It is recommended to conduct the exercise initially in Spanish, using the English version as a reference. Although it is not a literal translation, it maintains clinical and communicative equivalence and can serve as a guide for structuring the interview clearly and coherently.

This clinical case illustrates the importance of clearly explaining treatment options to the patient, considering their individual needs and preferences, in order to ensure informed decision-making and effective disease management.

| Historia Clínica | Medical History |
|---|---|
| La señora Rodríguez ha notado un aumento en el dolor y la inflamación en sus articulaciones de las manos, lo que ha afectado su capacidad para realizar actividades diarias. Ha tenido antecedentes de alergia a ciertos medicamentos, por lo que se evaluará cuidadosamente la tolerancia a los AINEs y se considerará el empleo de inhibidores selectivos de COX-2 si es necesario. | Mrs. Rodríguez has noticed a progressive increase in pain and inflammation in the joints of her hands, which has affected her ability to carry out daily activities. She has a history of allergies to certain medications, so her tolerance to NSAIDs will be carefully evaluated. In addition, the use of selective COX-2 inhibitors would be considered if deemed appropriate. |

| Discutiendo el manejo de la enfermedad | Discussing Disease Management |
|---|---|
| Médico: "Señora Rodríguez, ahora que hemos confirmado el diagnóstico de artritis reumatoide, vamos a discutir las opciones de tratamiento disponibles para usted. El objetivo del tratamiento es reducir la inflamación, aliviar el dolor y prevenir el daño articular a largo plazo." | Physician: "Mrs. Rodríguez, now that we have confirmed the diagnosis of rheumatoid arthritis, let's discuss the treatment options available to you. The goal of treatment is to reduce inflammation, relieve pain, and prevent long-term joint damage." |
| Paciente: "¿Qué tipos de tratamientos hay disponibles?". | Patient: "What types of treatments are available?". |
| Médico: "Hay varias opciones que podemos considerar. Primero, podemos iniciar con medicamentos antiinflamatorios no esteroideos (AINEs) para reducir el dolor y la inflamación. También podemos considerar medicamentos modificadores de la enfermedad (DMARDs) como el metotrexato, que pueden ayudar a ralentizar el progreso de la enfermedad, junto con ácido fólico para reducir efectos adversos y la realización de pruebas basales de función hepática y renal y hemograma, previo a su inicio." | Physician: "There are several options we can consider. First, we can start with nonsteroidal anti-inflammatory drugs (NSAIDs) to reduce pain and inflammation. We may also consider disease-modifying antirheumatic drugs (DMARDs), such as methotrexate, which can help slow the progression of the disease. Methotrexate is typically given with folic acid to minimize side effects, and we will need to perform baseline liver and kidney function tests, as well as a complete blood count, before starting." |
| Paciente: "He oído hablar de los medicamentos biológicos, ¿me podría explicar en qué consisten?". | Patient: "And what about biologic medications? I've heard of those." |

| Historia Clínica | Medical History |
|---|---|

Médico: "Los medicamentos biológicos son otra opción efectiva para tratar la artritis reumatoide. Funcionan bloqueando específicas moléculas involucradas en la inflamación. Sin embargo, suelen ser más costosos y pueden tener efectos secundarios específicos, por lo que los reservamos para pacientes que no responden bien a los DMARDs convencionales. En caso de respuesta subóptima al metotrexato, se considerarán agentes biológicos, previa evaluación de infecciones latentes como tuberculosis o hepatitis B."

Physician: "Biologic drugs are another effective option for treating rheumatoid arthritis. They work by targeting specific molecules involved in the inflammatory process. However, they are usually more expensive and may have specific side effects, so we reserve them for patients who do not respond well to conventional DMARDs. If your response to methotrexate is suboptimal, we will consider biological agents after screening for latent infections, such as tuberculosis or hepatitis B."

Paciente: ¿En cuanto a la terapia física o el estilo de vida, hay algo que deba hacer?"

Patient: "What about physical therapy and lifestyle changes?"

| Discutiendo el manejo de la enfermedad | Discussing Disease Management |
|---|---|

Médico: "La terapia física puede ser muy beneficiosa para mantener la movilidad y la fuerza en sus articulaciones. Además, hacer ejercicio regularmente, mantener un peso saludable y evitar el tabaquismo son medidas importantes para manejar su condición a largo plazo."

Physician: "Physical therapy can be very beneficial to help maintain joint mobility and muscle strength. In addition, regular exercise, maintaining a healthy weight, and avoiding smoking are important for long-term management of your condition."

| Plan de tratamiento | Treatment plan |
|---|---|

Medicamentos: Iniciar tratamiento con AINEs si no hay contraindicaciones; iniciar metotrexato como DMARD de primera línea, con suplementación de ácido fólico y monitoreo clínico y de laboratorios periódicos.

Medications: Start NSAIDs if there are no contraindications. Begin methotrexate as the first-line DMARD, with folic acid supplementation and periodic clinical and laboratory monitoring.

Terapia física: Referir a la paciente a un fisioterapeuta para desarrollar un programa de ejercicios personalizado, enfocado en la movilidad articular, fuerza muscular y adaptación funcional y a terapia ocupacional para preservación de la función de las manos.

Physical therapy: Refer the patient to a physical therapist to develop a personalized exercise program focused on joint mobility, muscle strength, and functional adaptation. Also refer to occupational therapy to support the preservation of hand function.

| Plan de tratamiento | Treatment plan |
|---|---|
| _Seguimiento_: _Citas regulares, inicialmente cada mes, para monitorear la respuesta al tratamiento, ajustar las dosis de los medicamentos según la respuesta clínica y la tolerancia, o para modificar la estrategia si es necesario._ | Follow-up: Monthly visits at the beginning of treatment to monitor therapeutic response, adjust medication dosages based on efficacy and tolerance, and revise the strategy if necessary. |
| _Educación: Proporcionar información sobre la enfermedad, manejo de síntomas y posibles complicaciones, especialmente osteoporosis y enfermedades cardiovasculares._ | Patient education: Provide information about the disease, symptom management, and potential complications, especially osteoporosis and cardiovascular disease. |

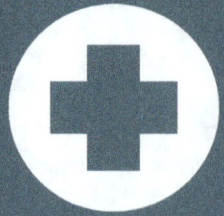

BOOK 5

# EFFECTIVE
# PATIENT EDUCATION
# IN SPANISH

### CLEAR HEALTHCARE INSTRUCTIONS FOR MEDICATION
### MANAGEMENT AND CHRONIC CONDITIONS.

ACQUIRE A LOT

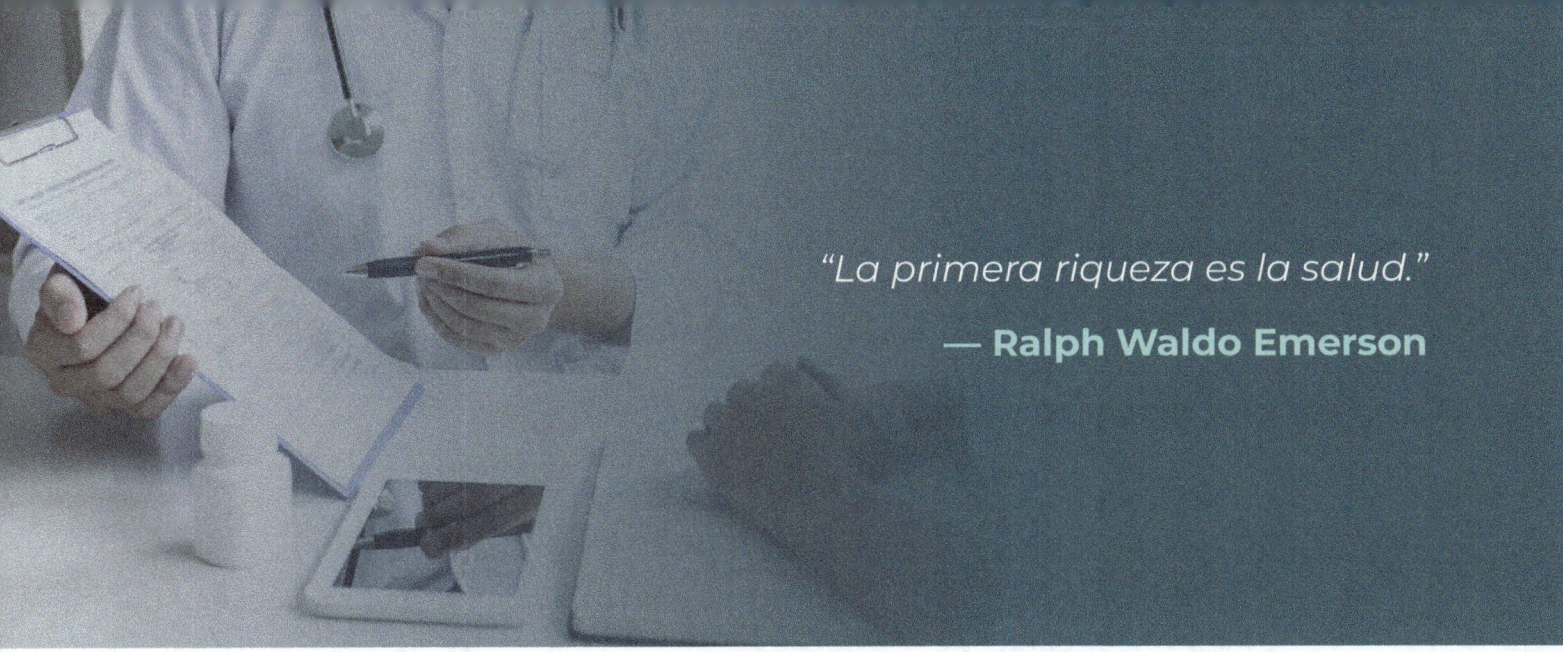

CHAPTER 10

# PROVIDING INSTRUCTIONS ON MEDICATION AND SELF-CARE

## 10.1 Giving Clear Instructions on How to Take Medications

Clear and effective communication about medication use is one of the most critical aspects of patient care. Patients must understand how, when, and why to take their medications to ensure adherence, maximize therapeutic benefits, and avoid potential complications. For Spanish-speaking patients, providing medication instructions in their native language not only enhances comprehension but also promotes safety and empowerment.

Healthcare providers should use clear, simple language that the patient can easily understand. Encouraging questions and verifying understanding can significantly improve medication compliance and health outcomes.

**1** **Explaining Dosage and Timing**

Specifically, when and how often the medication should be taken. Using plain language helps avoid misunderstandings.

Phrases you can use to explain this to the patient:

- *Tome esta pastilla con comida, dos veces al día.* — Take this pill with food twice a day.
- *Tome una cucharada de este jarabe cada 8 horas.* — *Take one tablespoon of this syrup every 8 hours.*
- *Tome una cápsula de este antibiótico cada 6 horas, iniciando (empezando) a las 6 a.m.* — Take one capsule of this antibiotic every 6 hours, starting at 6 a.m.

## 2  Stressing the Importance of Adherence

Explain the risks of skipping doses and reinforce the importance of taking medications as prescribed. It is essential that patients receiving treatment at home understand what to do if they forget to take a dose of their medication. Instructions should be clear, specific, and tailored to the type of medication, as some drugs can be taken as soon as the patient remembers, while others require waiting until the next scheduled dose. This helps prevent dangerous duplications or a decrease in the effectiveness of the treatment.

Phrases you can use to explain this to the patient:

- *No omita ninguna dosis.* — Do not skip any doses.
- *Si omite varias dosis, por favor comuníquelo a su médico.* — If you miss several doses, please inform your doctor.

## 3  Providing Guidance on Missed Doses

Patients should know what to do if they forget a dose. This helps prevent over- or under-medication.

Phrases you can use to explain this to the patient:

- *Si olvida una dosis, tómela tan pronto como lo recuerde.* — If you forget a dose, take it as soon as you remember.
- *Si olvida tomar una dosis de su antibiótico, tómela tan pronto como lo recuerde. Pero si ya casi es hora de la siguiente, omita la dosis olvidada y continúe con su horario regular. No tome dos dosis a la vez.* — If you forget to take a dose of your antibiotic, take it as soon as you remember. But if it's almost time for your next dose, skip the missed one and go back to your regular schedule. Do not take two doses at once.
- *Si se salta una dosis de su medicamento para la presión/tensión, no tome una dosis doble. Espere a la próxima toma y siga con su horario habitual. Avísele a su médico si olvida varias dosis.* — If you miss a dose of your blood pressure medication, do not take a double dose. Wait until your next scheduled dose and continue as usual. Let your doctor know if you miss multiple doses.

## 4  Best Practices for Clear Medication Communication

- Use teach-back methods to confirm understanding.
- Provide printed instructions in Spanish.
- Clarify if medication should be taken with or without food.
- Use visual aids or medication cards when appropriate.
- Encourage patients to keep a medication log or use reminders.

Giving clear medication instructions in Spanish is a simple but powerful way to improve adherence and outcomes. By ensuring that patients know how to take their medications correctly, providers help reduce errors and build patient confidence in managing their own care.

## 10.2 Explaining Potential Side Effects and What to Do

Telling patients about possible side effects helps them feel prepared and know when to ask for help. When patients are informed about what to expect and when to seek help, they are better equipped to manage their treatment and respond appropriately to complications.

For Spanish-speaking patients, this information must be presented in their preferred language to ensure full comprehension and reduce anxiety.

It's helpful to mention both common side effects and the rare, more serious ones—so the patient knows what to expect. Clarity and reassurance are key to helping patients feel prepared, rather than fearful.

### 1 Discussing Common Side Effects

Start by explaining mild or expected side effects so that patients are not alarmed if they occur.

Common useful  expressions

- *Este medicamento puede causar náuseas, por favor tómelo con las comidas* — This medication may cause nausea, please take it with food.

- *Este medicamento puede causarle somnolencia. Le recomiendo no conducir ni manejar (operar) maquinaria pesada mientras lo esté tomando. Si siente mucho sueño durante el día, es mejor tomarlo en la noche antes de dormir.* — This medication may cause drowsiness. I recommend that you don't drive or operate heavy machinery while taking it. If you feel very sleepy during the day, it's better to take it at night before going to bed.

- *Este medicamento puede causar irritación en el estómago. Le recomiendo tomarlo después de comer o con un vaso lleno de agua para reducir ese riesgo.* — This medication may cause stomach irritation. I recommend taking it after meals or with a full glass of water to reduce that risk.

### 2 Alerting Patients to Serious Symptoms

Describe symptoms that require immediate medical attention and advise patients to seek emergency care if they occur.

Phrases you can use to say this effectively:

- *Si nota sarpullido, picazón, dificultad para respirar o hinchazón en la cara o los labios después de tomar este medicamento, suspenda su uso y acuda de inmediato a un servicio de urgencias.* — If you notice a rash, itching, trouble breathing, or swelling of the face or lips after taking this medication, stop taking it and go to the emergency room immediately.

- *Este medicamento puede afectar el hígado. Si nota coloración amarilla en la piel o en los ojos, orina oscura, náuseas intensas o cansancio inusual, suspenda el medicamento y consulte al médico de inmediato.* — This medication can affect your liver. If you notice yellowing of your skin or eyes, dark urine, severe nausea, or unusual fatigue, stop taking the medication and contact your doctor immediately.

**3** **Encouraging Communication About Side Effects**

Let patients know that they should report any side effects—especially those that are new, persistent, or unexpected.

For this, you can use the following phrase:

*Si nota cualquier cambio en su cuerpo después de tomar este medicamento, por favor infórmeselo a su médico, sin demora. No dude en hablar; su opinión es clave para su tratamiento.* — If you notice any changes in your body after taking this medication, please inform your doctor. Don't hesitate to speak up; your input is essential to your care.

**4** **Best Practices for Discussing Side Effects**

- Explain both common and serious side effects clearly.
- Provide written materials in Spanish listing side effects and emergency symptoms.
- Use patient-friendly language to avoid causing unnecessary fear.
- Reassure patients that side effects are manageable and often temporary.
- Make sure patients know when and how to contact their provider.

When patients understand the potential side effects of their medications, they can act quickly and responsibly if a reaction occurs. Spanish-speaking patients deserve the same level of clarity and reassurance, making linguistic and cultural sensitivity essential in these discussions. Initiative-taking communication about side effects empowers patients to take part fully in their own care.

## 10.3 Providing Guidance on Wound Care and Hygiene

Effective wound care and personal hygiene are critical components of post-treatment recovery. Proper instructions help patients avoid complications such as infections, delayed healing, or the need for further medical intervention. When communicating with Spanish-speaking patients, healthcare professionals must provide clear, culturally respectful guidance using accessible language.

By ensuring that patients understand how to care for their wounds and maintain hygiene, clinicians support faster healing, reduce emergency visits, and improve patient satisfaction and outcomes.

## 1 Cleaning and Taking care of the Wound

Instruct patients on how to clean the wound and explain its importance (to remove debris and bacteria). Use plain language and encourage gentle handling. Teach them how to recognize signs of infection. Always emphasize that consistent wound care promotes faster healing and reduces the risk of complications.

How to word it

- *Lave la herida con agua y jabón suave todos los días. — Wash the wound with water and mild soap daily.*

- *Los siguientes son signos de alarma por posible infección: enrojecimiento, hinchazón, calor local, presencia de pus o aumento del dolor. Consulte a su médico si presenta alguno de ellos* — The following are warning signs of a possible infection: redness, swelling, warmth at the site, presence of pus, or increased pain. Contact your doctor if you experience any of them.

- *No es necesario que descubra la herida, la revisaremos en la próxima consulta en 5 días. —* You don't need to uncover the wound; we will check it at your next appointment in 5 days

## 2 Keeping the Area Clean and Dry

Explain that a clean and dry environment prevents bacterial growth and reduces the risk of infection.

How to word it:

- *Mantenga el área de la herida limpia y seca. — Keep the area clean and dry.*

- *Mantenga la incisión cubierta durante 48 horas. Si necesita ducharse, cúbrala con un plástico completamente impermeable. Después del baño, séquela con toques suaves, sin frotar. —* Keep the incision covered for 48 hours. If you need to shower, cover it with a completely waterproof plastic covering. After bathing, gently pat it dry without rubbing.

## 3 Changing the Bandage Properly

Provide instructions on how often and how to change the dress. Emphasize the importance of following these instructions exactly.

How to word it:

- *Cambie el vendaje según las indicaciones. — Change the bandage as instructed.*

- *No utilice vendajes previamente usados. — Do not reuse old bandages.*

- *Lávese bien las manos antes y después de cambiar el vendaje para evitar infecciones. — Wash your hands thoroughly before and after changing the bandage to prevent infection.*

## 4 Additional Tips for Successful Healing

When patients understand how to care for their wounds, they can feel more confident and in control of their recovery For Spanish-speaking patients, using appropriate language and confirming understanding helps ensure compliance and reduce complications. Effective communication in this area is a vital part of holistic and patient-centered care.

Below, you will find the key wound care tips translated into Spanish, ready to be shared directly with patients.

- ⊙ *Evite tocar la herida con las manos sin lavar.* — Avoid touching the wound with unwashed hands.

- ⊙ *Lave sus manos con agua y jabón antes y después de manipular la herida.* — Wash your hands with water and soap before and after handling the wound.

- ⊙ *Vigile los signos de infección: Calor local, enrojecimiento, edema (hinchazón), pus o fiebre.* — Watch for signs of infection: redness, swelling, pus, or fever.

- ⊙ *Evite mojar la herida a menos que se le indique.* — Avoid soaking the wound unless instructed.

- ⊙ *Acuda a sus citas de control para revisar la herida.* — Keep follow-up appointments for wound checks.

- ⊙ *Avise al personal de salud cualquier preocupación que tenga.* — Notify your healthcare provider of any concerns.

## 10.4 Instructing Patients on Dietary Modifications and Lifestyle Changes

Even small changes in diet and daily habits can make a big difference in managing health conditions, especially chronic ones. This guidance is most effective when it is tailored to the patient's cultural background, daily habits, and health goals. In Spanish-speaking clinical settings, providing instructions in the patient's language fosters clarity, motivation, and long-term adherence.

### 1 Dietary Modifications

Nutrition plays a significant role in managing conditions such as diabetes, hypertension, and cardiovascular disease. Patients should receive realistic, culturally relevant advice on improving their diet.

Phrases you can use to encourage this behavior :

- ⊙ *Necesita reducir el consumo de sal y los alimentos procesados.* — *You need to reduce your intake of salt and processed foods.*

- ⊙ *Evite las sodas / gaseosas / refrescos regulares o dietéticas.* — Avoid both regular and diet sodas / soft drinks.

- ⊙ *Evite el consumo de azúcares. Si desea endulzar sus bebidas emplee endulzantes a base de stevia.* — Avoid sugar consumption. If you wish to sweeten, use stevia-based sweeteners.

## 2  Encouraging Physical Activity

Regular physical activity supports weight management, cardiovascular health, and mental well-being. Even small, consistent changes can yield significant benefits.

Phrases you can use to encourage this behavior :

- *Camine al menos 30 minutos al día.* — Walk at least 30 minutes a day.
- *Realice ejercicio al menos 3 veces por semana, durante mínimo 30 minutos cada vez.* — Engage in exercise at least 3 times a week for a minimum of 30 minutes each session.
- *Aproveche cualquier momento del día para aumentar su actividad física. Por ejemplo, subir escaleras en lugar de usar ascensores o escaleras mecánicas.* — Use any opportunity during the day to increase your physical activity, such as taking the stairs instead of elevators or escalators.

## 3  Reducing Harmful Habits

Tobacco and excessive alcohol consumption are major risk factors for many health conditions. Encourage behavior changes while offering support and resources.

Phrases you can use to encourage this behavior :

- *Deje de fumar y limite el consumo de alcohol.* — Quit smoking and limit alcohol consumption.
- *Reduzca sus niveles de ansiedad y estrés, medite, haga caminatas o haga yoga.* — Reduce your levels of anxiety and stress — try meditation, walking, or yoga.
- *Tenga comidas con porciones de menor tamaño.* — Have meals with smaller portions.

## 4  Best Practices for Health Counseling

- Use specific, achievable goals (e.g., walk 30 minutes daily).
- Reinforce changes at each follow-up appointment.
- Provide written handouts in Spanish with clear instructions.
- Respect cultural food practices and suggest alternatives when necessary.
- Acknowledge the patient's efforts and provide encouragement.

Empowering patients to make dietary and lifestyle changes requires empathy, respect, and education. By delivering clear, culturally appropriate instructions in Spanish, healthcare professionals can build trust, increase compliance, and improve health outcomes in diverse patient populations.

## 10.5 Explaining the Importance of Follow-Up Appointments

Follow-up appointments are essential for evaluating patient progress, monitoring treatment effectiveness, and adjusting care plans as needed. These visits ensure continuity of care and provide an opportunity to address any new concerns or side effects. For Spanish-speaking patients, communicating the value of these appointments clearly and respectfully reinforces engagement and trust.

### 1 Why Follow-Up Matters

Explain that follow-up visits are not just routine, they are a vital part of personalized care. Reassure patients that their purpose is to support their recovery and health.

Model phrases you can use:

- *Es importante que asista a sus controles programados para evaluar su progreso.* — It's important that you attend your scheduled follow-up appointments to monitor your progress.

- *Después de una cirugía, es muy importante asistir a sus controles programados para verificar que la herida esté cicatrizando correctamente y detectar cualquier signo de complicación a tiempo.* — After surgery, it's very important to attend your scheduled follow-up appointments to ensure the wound is healing properly and to catch any signs of complications early.

- *Puesto que está en tratamiento con anticoagulantes orales, asistir a sus controles programados es fundamental para ajustar la dosis y prevenir efectos adversos o complicaciones.* — Since you are on oral anticoagulant therapy, attending your scheduled follow-up appointments is essential to adjust the dosage and prevent adverse effects or complications.

### 2 Providing Clear Scheduling Information

Always confirm the date and time of the next appointment. Provide written instructions when possible.

Appropriate wording:

- *Su próxima cita es en dos semanas.* — Your next appointment is in two weeks.

- *Por favor, llame a la clínica un mes antes para confirmar la fecha exacta de su próxima cita.* — Please call the clinic one month in advance to confirm the exact date of your next appointment.

- *Llame unos días antes de su cita para recibir indicaciones sobre qué debe traer.* — Call a few days before your appointment to receive instructions about what to bring.

- *Si no puede asistir, por favor comuníquese con nosotros al menos 24 horas antes para reprogramar su cita.* — If you are unable to attend, please contact us at least 24 hours in advance to reschedule your appointment.

### 3 Encouraging Communication

Let patients know they can reach out with questions or to reschedule if needed. This helps reduce no-shows and promotes open communication.

Appropriate wording:

- *Llámenos si tiene alguna pregunta.* — Call if you have any questions.

- *Es muy importante para mí que usted entienda toda la información. Puede preguntarme cuantas veces necesite.* — It's very important to me that you understand all the information. Feel free to ask me as many times as you need.

- *A veces las personas mayores no quieren molestar, pero para mí es muy importante saber cómo se siente. Si algo le incomoda, por favor hágamelo saber.* — Sometimes older adults don't want to be a bother, but it's very important for me to know how you're feeling. If something is bothering you, please let me know.

**4** **Best Practices for Follow-Up Engagement**

- Provide the appointment details both verbally and in writing.
- Explain the specific purpose of the follow-up visit.
- Reiterate the importance of returning even if the patient feels better.
- Encourage questions and reassure the patient that follow-up is part of good care.
- Offer culturally appropriate reminders and accommodation if needed.

Ensuring that patients understand the purpose and timing of follow-up appointments strengthens care continuity and outcomes. When instructions are delivered clearly and respectfully in Spanish, patients are more likely to stay engaged in their care plan and communicate openly about their health.

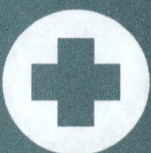

## CHAPTER 11

# COMMUNICATING IN PRIMARY CARE SETTINGS

### 11.1 Addressing Common Acute Illnesses (Colds, Flu, Infections)

Effective communication is critical when addressing common acute illnesses in primary care, such as colds, the flu, and minor infections. These conditions often cause patient anxiety, even though they are typically self-limiting. For Spanish-speaking patients, clear symptom-focused language and reassurance can greatly improve understanding, satisfaction, and adherence to treatment plans.

**1  Gathering Key Symptoms**

Ask specific questions to identify the nature and severity of the illness. Clear questions in Spanish help patients describe symptoms more accurately.

Useful phrases in specific clinical scenarios:

*Paciente con neumopatía* **/ Patient with lung disease:**

- ⊙ *¿Han reaparecido la fiebre, la tos o el dolor al respirar?* — Have the fever, cough, or pain when breathing?

*Paciente con cáncer /* **Cancer patient**:

- ⊙ *¿Ha notado nuevos síntomas desde la última cita, como fatiga intensa, dolor persistente o pérdida de apetito? Es importante que me cuente cualquier cambio, por pequeño que parezca.* — Have you noticed any new symptoms since your last visit, such as severe fatigue, persistent pain, or loss of appetite? Please let me know any changes, no matter how small they may seem.

*Paciente trasplantado /* **Transplant patient**:

- ⊙  *¿Ha sentido fiebre, escalofríos, dolor en la zona del trasplante o algún cambio en su energía o apetito?* — Have you experienced fever, chills, pain around the transplant site, or any changes in your energy level or appetite?

*Paciente con enfermedad renal crónica /* **Patient with Chronic Kidney Disease**:

- *¿Ha tenido hinchazón en las piernas, dificultad para respirar, picazón en la piel o cambios en la orina? Necesito saberlo para ajustar su tratamiento si es necesario.* — Have you had swelling in your legs, shortness of breath, itchy skin, or changes in your urine? I need to know so we can adjust your treatment if needed.

*Niño con diarrea /* **Child with diarrhea**:

- *¿Desde hace cuántos días tiene diarrea? ¿Ha notado (observado) sangre, moco o mal olor? ¿Está comiendo bien? ¿Ha bajado de peso o parece más cansado de lo normal?* — How many days has the diarrhea lasted? Have you noticed any blood, mucus, or foul odor? Is the child eating well? Has there been any weight loss or does the child seem more tired than usual?

## 2  Explaining Likely Causes

Patients often worry about the seriousness of their symptoms. Explaining the probable cause helps them understand the situation and what to expect.

Appropriate wording:

- *Es probable que tenga una infección viral.* — You likely have a viral infection.

- *El dolor que siente puede deberse a una sobrecarga muscular o a un esfuerzo físico reciente. Es común que los músculos se inflamen o duelan después de una actividad intensa.* — The pain you're experiencing may be due to muscle overuse or recent physical exertion. It's common for muscles to become sore or inflamed after intense activity

- *Sus síntomas podrían estar relacionados con una reacción del sistema inmunológico, donde el cuerpo ataca por error sus propios tejidos. Esto ocurre en algunas enfermedades autoinmunes.* — Your symptoms may be related to an immune system reaction, where the body mistakenly attacks its own tissues. This happens in some autoimmune conditions

## 3  Recommending Symptom Relief

Provide simple and effective recommendations, including medications and home remedies. Clarify that viral infections typically don't require antibiotics.

Model phrases you can use

- *Vamos a recetarle algo para aliviar los síntomas.* — We'll prescribe something to relieve your symptoms.

- *Para aliviar el dolor lumbar, le recomiendo aplicar compresas calientes dos veces al día y evitar levantar objetos pesados. También puede realizar estiramientos suaves si no le causan molestias.* — To relieve lower back pain, I recommend applying warm compresses twice a day and avoiding heavy lifting. Gentle stretching can also help, as long as it doesn't cause discomfort.

- *Para reducir la acidez, evite comidas muy grasosas o picantes, y procure no acostarse justo después de comer. Comer porciones pequeñas varias veces al día también puede ayudar.* — To reduce heartburn, avoid greasy or spicy foods, and try not to lie down right after eating. Eating small meals throughout the day may also help."

- ⊙ *Dado que presenta dolor frecuente y la hernia es visible, lo más recomendable es una cirugía. Es un procedimiento común y generalmente ambulatorio.* — Since you're experiencing frequent pain and the hernia is noticeable, a surgery is the best option. It's a common and typically outpatient procedure."

### 4  Best Practices for Acute Illness Encounters

- ⊙ Use language that normalizes symptoms and reduces fear.
- ⊙ Educate patients about the expected course of the illness.
- ⊙ Emphasize rest, hydration, and symptom monitoring.
- ⊙ Clarify when to return or seek further care (e.g., worsening symptoms or prolonged fever).
- ⊙ Offer written care instructions in Spanish.

In primary care, effective communication about acute illnesses builds patient confidence and ensures safe, appropriate treatment. By using accurate, empathetic Spanish-language communication, healthcare professionals can foster better outcomes and reduce unnecessary antibiotic use.

## 11.2 Managing Chronic Conditions (Diabetes, Hypertension, Asthma)

Chronic conditions such as diabetes, hypertension, and asthma are among the most common health challenges seen in primary care. Managing these conditions requires ongoing communication, patient education, and proactive care planning. For Spanish-speaking patients, culturally competent conversations that encourage involvement in their own care are essential to improving health outcomes.

### 1  Emphasizing the Importance of Control

Patients must understand the importance of consistently managing their diseases, especially chronic ones, to avoid serious complications. Always provide education, reinforce the treatment goals, and acknowledge the patient's progress and achievements.

You might say:

- ⊙ *Necesitamos controlar su presión arterial y nivel de azúcar.* — We need to control your blood pressure and blood sugar.

- ⊙ *Controlar su colesterol y triglicéridos es clave para proteger su corazón y prevenir infartos o problemas circulatorios. Coma saludable, haga ejercicio y tome su medicación lo ayudará a mantener una buena salud cardiovascular."* — Managing your cholesterol and triglycerides is essential for protecting your heart and preventing heart attacks or circulation problems. Eating a healthy diet, staying physically active, and taking your medications as prescribed will help you maintain good cardiovascular health.

- *Mantener su asma bajo control le permite respirar mejor y evitar visitas a urgencias. Para lograrlo procure usar sus inhaladores correctamente.* — Keeping your asthma under control helps you breathe better and avoid emergency room visits. To achieve this, take care to use your inhalers correctly.

## 2 Encouraging Medication Adherence

Non-adherence is one of the leading causes of poor chronic disease control. Ask direct but respectful questions to assess consistency, explore the patient's reasons, and address them appropriately.

You might say:

- *¿Está tomando sus medicamentos regularmente?* — Are you taking your medications regularly?

- *A veces es difícil seguir el tratamiento todos los días. ¿Hay algo que le esté impidiendo tomar sus medicamentos como se indicó?* — Sometimes it's hard to follow a treatment every day. Is there anything that's making it difficult for you to take your medications as prescribed?"

## 3 Preventing Complications Through Education

Explain how consistent care—including a balanced diet, appropriate physical activity, medication adherence, and regular follow-up appointments—helps maintain stability, reduce symptoms, and prevent emergency visits or hospitalizations. When patients understand the "why" behind their treatment plan, they are more likely to take an active role in managing their condition.

Education not only improves their understanding of health, but also empowers patients to make informed decisions, recognize warning signs, and seek timely care—ultimately leading to a better quality of life and reduced healthcare costs.

Example Phrases:

- *Cuidarse cada día es la mejor forma de evitar complicaciones graves en el futuro.* —Taking care of yourself every day is the best way to prevent serious problems in the future.

- *Puede disminuir sus ingresos por urgencias si sigue su tratamiento y asiste a sus controles.* —You can reduce your emergency room visits if you follow your treatment and attend your check-ups.

## 4 Best Practices for Chronic Disease Communication
- Provide clear explanations of disease processes and goals.
- Use visuals and translated materials when possible.
- Reinforce the need for regular follow-up visits and lab tests.
- Discuss lifestyle changes alongside medications.
- Involve family members or caregivers if appropriate.

Managing chronic conditions effectively in Spanish-speaking patients requires more than medical expertise—it demands empathy, education, and a commitment to communication. Helping patients take control of their health through consistent dialogue fosters long-term stability and better quality of life.

## 11.3 Providing Preventative Care Advice (Vaccinations, Screenings)

Preventative care is a cornerstone of primary care medicine. It involves anticipating potential health issues and addressing them before symptoms arise. This initiative-taking approach includes vaccinations, routine screenings, and patient education. For Spanish-speaking patients, it is especially important to convey the purpose and value of preventative care in accessible, culturally sensitive language.

### 1 Discussing Vaccination Status

Vaccinations protect individuals and communities from serious diseases, both in adults and children. Providers should routinely check if patients are up to date and explain why certain vaccines are important. It is also essential to explore why a patient has not received a recommended vaccine, in order to identify and address any doubts, fears, or access barriers that may be preventing them from completing their immunization schedule.

Example phrases to discuss vaccination status:

- *¿Está al día con sus vacunas?* — Are you up to date on your vaccinations?

- *¿Podría contarme si hay alguna razón por la que no vacunó a su hijo?* — Could you tell me if there's any reason why your child hasn't been vaccinated?

- *¿Podría contarme la razón de su prevención a ser vacunado?* —Could you share with me what's made you hesitant about getting vaccinated?

### 2 Recommending Routine Screenings

Age-appropriate screenings, such as mammograms and colonoscopies, play a key role in early detection. Providers should explain the recommended timeline and reassure patients about the process.

Phrases you can use to explain this to the patient:

- *Recomendamos una mamografía / colonoscopía según su edad.* — We recommend a mammogram / colonoscopy based on your age.

- *A partir de los 50 años (o antes si hay antecedentes familiares), es importante que los hombres se realicen chequeos de próstata, que pueden incluir el examen del antígeno prostático específico (PSA) y el tacto rectal.* — Starting at age 50 (or earlier with a family history), it's important for men to have prostate screenings, which may include a PSA blood test and a digital rectal exam.

- *Los adultos mayores deben realizarse exámenes visuales de forma regular para detectar problemas como cataratas, glaucoma o degeneración macular. Incluso si no presentan síntomas, el examen periódico es esencial.* — Older adults should have regular eye exams to detect issues like cataracts, glaucoma, or macular degeneration. Even if they have no symptoms, regular eye exams are essential.

- *Tanto la presión arterial como la glucemia deben controlarse con regularidad, incluso si usted se siente bien. La hipertensión y la diabetes pueden no presentar síntomas al inicio, pero si no se detectan a tiempo pueden causar complicaciones graves.* —Both blood pressure and blood sugar should be checked regularly, even if you feel fine. High blood pressure and diabetes may not cause symptoms early on, but if left undetected, they can lead to serious complications.

### 3  Explaining the Purpose of Preventative Tests

Patients may hesitate to undergo screenings without symptoms. Emphasize that the goal is to detect disease early when it is most treatable.

These are some common ways to do this:

- *Estas pruebas pueden detectar problemas antes de que aparezcan los síntomas.* — These tests can detect problems before they cause symptoms.

- *Estas pruebas permiten evaluar su estado de salud general y conocer si tiene factores de riesgo para ciertas enfermedades. Con esa información, usted y su equipo médico pueden tomar decisiones informadas sobre su cuidado.* — These tests help assess your overall health and identify whether you have risk factors for certain diseases. With that information, you and your healthcare team can make informed decisions about your care.

- *Estas pruebas, la presión arterial y la glicemia, ayudan a prevenir enfermedades cardiovasculares, renales y otras enfermedades crónicas.* — These screenings, blood pressure and blood sugar, can help prevent cardiovascular disease, kidney problems, and other chronic conditions.

### 4  Best Practices for Preventative Care Conversations

- Normalize routine care as part of staying healthy.
- Provide written schedules for screenings and vaccines.
- Address myths or concerns about vaccines or procedures.
- Personalize advice based on patient age, sex, and risk factors.
- Reinforce that prevention is often easier and less costly than treatment.

Preventative care empowers patients to take charge of their health. Clear, initiative-taking communication in Spanish helps ensure patients follow through with recommended tests and immunizations, ultimately improving long-term outcomes and reducing health disparities.

## 11.4 Discussing Mental Health Concerns

Mental health is a fundamental component of overall well-being. However, for many Spanish-speaking patients, discussing emotional or psychological concerns can be challenging due to stigma, cultural beliefs, or lack of access to appropriate resources. Healthcare providers must approach these conversations with empathy, cultural competence, and clear, accessible language to foster trust and open dialogue, even if it takes several visits to help the patient open up and share information.

### 1  Initiating the Conversation

Gently opening the door to discuss mental health can help normalize the topic. Using open-ended questions allows patients to share their experiences without feeling judged.

Model phrases for doing this include:

- *A veces, el estrés o las emociones pueden afectar nuestra salud. ¿Cómo se ha sentido últimamente, en cuanto a su estado de ánimo o sus emociones?* — Sometimes stress or emotions can affect our health. How have you been feeling lately, in terms of your mood or emotions?

- *¿Ha sentido tristeza, ansiedad o falta de motivación últimamente?* — Have you felt sadness, anxiety, or lack of motivation recently?

### 2  Reducing Stigma and Offering Support

Assure patients that mental health is a normal and treatable aspect of health. Expressing understanding and support encourages patients to speak openly.

Here are some common ways to do this:

- *Hablar de su salud mental es importante. Estoy aquí para usted, no está solo(a).* — Talking about your mental health matters. I'm here for you — you're not alone.

- *Hablar de lo que uno siente no es una señal de debilidad, sino un paso valiente hacia el bienestar. Estoy aquí para acompañarlo(a) y apoyarlo(a).* — Talking about your feelings isn't a sign of weakness. It's a brave step toward healing. I'm here to support and walk with you.

### 3  Offering Resources and Referrals

If a patient expresses concerns, provide information about available mental health services, including psychologists, counselors, or community resources. Offer referrals with sensitivity and empower the patient to take the next step.

Here are some common ways to do this:

- *No todos saben que existen servicios para hablar con alguien sobre lo que sienten. Si quiere, puedo contarle qué opciones hay.* — Not everyone knows there are services where you can talk to someone about how you feel. If you'd like, I can share what's available.

- *A veces, la familia no entiende lo que estamos pasando. Pero buscar ayuda externa también es una forma de cuidarse.* — Sometimes families don't understand what we're going through, but getting outside help is also a way to care for yourself.

- *A veces, las preocupaciones emocionales están relacionadas con situaciones difíciles en casa o en el entorno. ¿Hay algo que le esté afectando últimamente y que desee compartir? — Sometimes emotional concerns are connected to difficult situations at home or in your surroundings. Is there anything affecting you lately that you'd like to talk about?*

Emotional symptoms can be a warning sign. Beyond their clinical presentation, it is essential to recognize that a patient's emotional distress may be linked to deep or traumatic personal experiences. For this reason, the approach should go beyond the surface and sensitively consider potential psychosocial factors at play.

Always explore underlying causes of emotional distress. In all cases where a patient presents signs of emotional distress, it is essential to explore the potential presence of interpersonal or domestic violence, abuse, or other psychosocial stressors that may be contributing to their condition. These underlying factors are often not disclosed voluntarily and require a safe, respectful, and culturally sensitive environment to be uncovered.

Engaging interdisciplinary support—such as social workers, psychologists, or behavioral health specialists—can be extremely valuable in identifying the root causes of the patient's emotional state. These professionals can assist in conducting more in-depth assessments, facilitating disclosure, and providing appropriate interventions or referrals.

Remember: Emotional symptoms may reflect not only mental health conditions but also adverse life circumstances that require coordinated and compassionate care.

### 4 Best Practices for Mental Health Conversations

- Create a safe, nonjudgmental space for discussion.
- Acknowledge the validity of emotional concerns.
- Be mindful of language and cultural values.
- Normalize mental health check-ins as part of routine care.
- Provide reassurance that help is available and recovery is possible.

Addressing mental health in primary care settings is a vital step toward whole-person care. By using respectful Spanish-language communication and culturally sensitive practices, providers can reduce barriers, build trust, and guide patients toward the support they need.

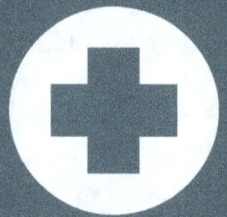

BOOK 6

# ADVANCED HEALTHCARE COMMUNICATION IN SPANISH

## A GUIDE FOR MEDICAL SPECIALTIES, EMERGENCY CARE, AND CULTURALLY COMPETENT PATIENT COUNSELING

ACQUIRE A LOT

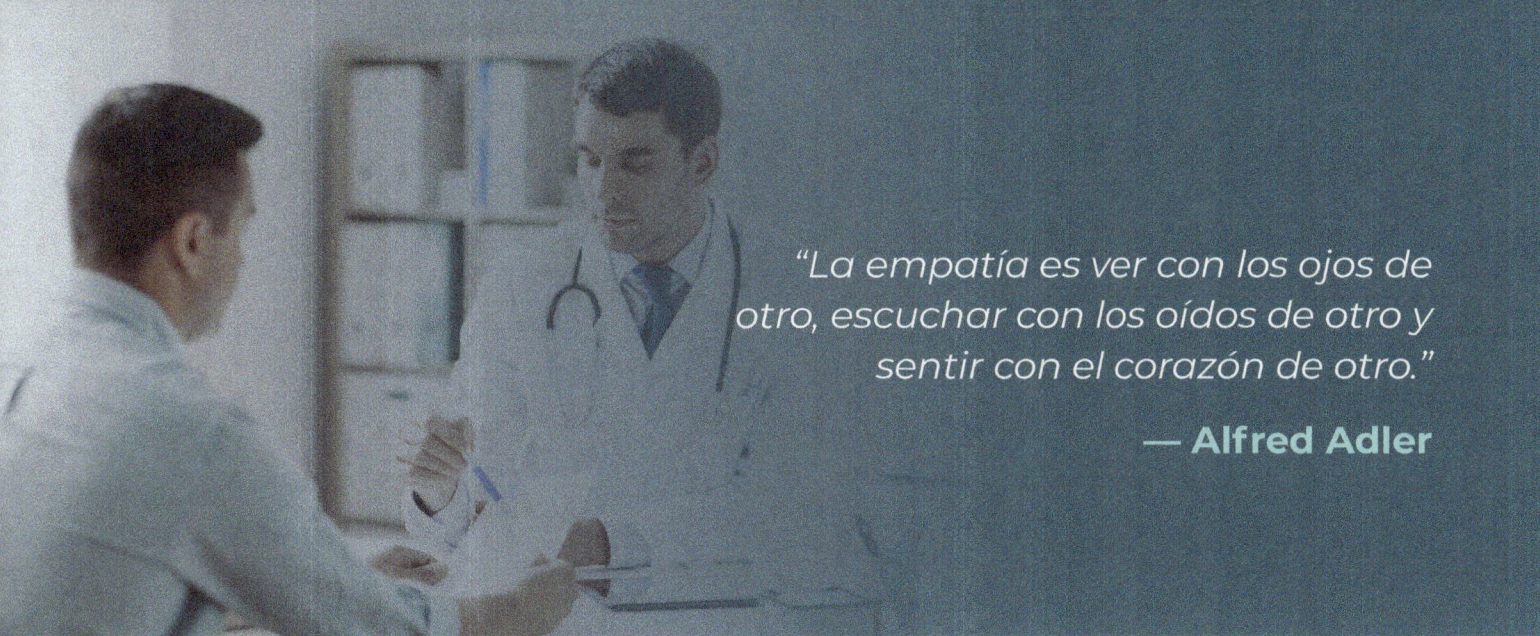

*"La empatía es ver con los ojos de otro, escuchar con los oídos de otro y sentir con el corazón de otro."*

**— Alfred Adler**

## CHAPTER 12

# COMMUNICATING IN EMERGENCY MEDICINE

## 12.1 Rapid Assessment and Triage: Asking Crucial Questions Quickly

In emergency medicine, rapid and effective communication can mean the difference between life and death. In these high-stakes situations, misunderstandings can have serious consequences. Communicating effectively in urgent or emergency settings requires clarity, composure, and efficiency.

Spanish-speaking patients may arrive at the emergency department with urgent symptoms, pain, or confusion, and providers must act swiftly to assess the situation while building trust and understanding. This section focuses on the essential Spanish-language questions and communication strategies used during triage and initial evaluation.

**1  Initiating Rapid Assessment**

The first moments of contact are critical for assessing the patient's level of consciousness, vital signs, and chief complaint. Clear, direct questions help identify life-threatening issues quickly. Use gestures or body language when needed to enhance understanding. Always check for comprehension, especially if the patient appears confused or afraid and use short, clear sentences and avoid medical jargon.

Example Phrases:

- *¿Qué pasó* — What happened?
- *¿Puede decirme qué pasó?* —  Can you tell me what happened?
- *¿Está sangrando? ¿Por dónde? ¿Desde hace cuánto?* — Are you bleeding? From where? Since when?

- *¿Tiene dolor en el pecho o dificultad para respirar?* — Do you have chest pain or trouble breathing?
- *¿Dónde le duele?* — Where does it hurt?
- *¿Ha perdido el conocimiento o se ha caído?* — Have you lost consciousness or had a fall?
- *¿Está vomitando, tiene diarrea intensa o fiebre alta sin mejoría?* — Are you experiencing vomiting, severe diarrhea, or a high fever that hasn't improved?
- *¿Está tomando algún medicamento importante que haya omitido hoy?* — Are you taking any important medications that you missed today?
- *¿Ha sufrido una herida o golpe?* — Do you have a wound or injury?

## 2  Gathering Critical Medical Information

Essential medical history—such as current medications, allergies, and chronic conditions—should be gathered promptly to inform safe treatment and avoid complications.

Model phrases :

- *¿Está tomando algún medicamento? ¿Tiene alguna alergia?* — Are you taking any medication or have allergies?
- *¿Cómo ha estado su presión / azúcar / respiración en los últimos días?* —How has your blood pressure / blood sugar / breathing been over the last few days?
- *¿Tiene alguna condición médica importante, como diabetes o hipertensión?* — Do you have any major medical conditions such as diabetes or high blood pressure?
- *¿Ha podido tomar sus medicamentos como se los indicaron?* — Have you been able to take your medications as prescribed?
- *¿Ha tenido que ir a urgencias, hospitalizarse o consultar otro médico en las últimas semanas?* — Have you needed to go to the ER, been hospitalized, or seen another doctor in the past few weeks?
- *¿Le han practicado recientemente alguna cirugía o procedimiento?* — Have you recently had any surgery or medical procedure?

## 3  Clarifying Symptoms and Severity

Assessing the onset, duration, and severity of symptoms provides crucial diagnostic information. The language must be simple and clear, especially under stress or when the patient is in pain.

Useful expressions when collecting patient information:

- *¿Cuándo comenzaron los síntomas?* — When did the symptoms start?
- *¿El dolor es constante o va y viene?* — Is the pain constant or does it come and go?
- *¿Cómo calificaría el dolor del uno al diez?* — How would you rate the pain from one to ten?
- *¿Los síntomas han cambiado desde que comenzaron?* — Have the symptoms changed since they started?

- *¿Ha notado que los síntomas empeoran en algún momento del día o con alguna actividad?* — Have you noticed if the symptoms get worse at any particular time of day or with certain activities?

### 4 Ensuring Understanding and Cooperation

It is important to maintain calm, supportive communication. Even in high-stress situations, providers should reassure the patient and ensure they understand the next steps.

Effective phrasing:

- *Trate de relajarse mientras lo examinamos.* — *Try to relax while we examine you.*
- *¿Le quedó claro lo que debe hacer ahora? ¿Hay algo que quisiera que le explique de nuevo?* — Is everything clear about what you need to do now? Is there anything you'd like me to explain again?
- *¿Está de acuerdo con el plan del que hemos hablado?* — Are you okay with the plan we've discussed?
- *Si tiene alguna duda ahora o más adelante, o algo cambia, por favor no dude en llamarnos.* — If you have any questions now or later, or if anything changes, please don't hesitate to call us.

Effective emergency communication relies on clarity, compassion, and cultural awareness. Using focused Spanish-language questions during triage helps providers deliver timely, life-saving care while ensuring that patients feel heard, safe, and understood.

## 12.2 Giving Urgent Instructions to Patients and Family Members

In emergency settings, time is of the essence and clear communication can save lives. Healthcare professionals must issue direct, respectful, and understandable instructions—especially when working with Spanish-speaking patients and their families. In high-pressure situations, communication must remain calm, yet firm, ensuring that patients feel safe and that clinical care proceeds without interference.

### 1 Giving Immediate Instructions to Patients

When a patient's condition is critical, concise instructions can help prevent further harm. These phrases should be delivered with a steady tone and reinforced with visual cues or gestures when possible.

How to word it:

- *¡No se mueva! Vamos a ayudarle.* — Don't move! We are going to help you.
- *No se mueva, podría empeorar la lesión.* — Don't move, it could make the injury worse.
- *Respire profundamente y con calma.* — Breathe deeply and calmly.
- *No hable, solo respire despacio.* — Don't speak, just breathe slowly.

- *Trate de quedarse quieto mientras lo examinamos.* — Try to stay still while we examine you.
- *¡Mantenga los ojos abiertos y míreme!* — Keep your eyes open and look at me.

## 2  Addressing Family Members and Bystanders

Family members are often present in emergency situations and may feel helpless or anxious. Providing them with clear instructions helps reduce confusion and enables healthcare teams to work efficiently.

Appropriate wording:

- *Por favor, acompáñenos a la sala de emergencias.* — Please come with us to the emergency room.
- *Necesitamos espacio para trabajar; manténganse atrás.* — We need space to work; please stay back.
- *Uno de ustedes puede acompañarnos. Los demás deben esperar aquí.* — One of you may come with us. The others need to wait here.
- *¿Es usted un familiar cercano o su representante legal?* — Are you a close family member or the patient's legal representative?
- *Mantenga la calma, estamos haciendo todo lo posible.* — Please stay calm, we're doing everything we can.
- *¿Tiene el paciente alguna condición médica que debamos saber?* — Does the patient have any medical condition we should know about?
- *Le explicaremos lo que está pasando en cuanto podamos.* — We'll explain what's happening as soon as we can.
- *Uno de ustedes, por favor, explíqueme qué ha ocurrido.* — One of you, please tell me what happened.

## 3  Reassurance in High-Stress Moments

Even in moments of crisis, a few reassuring words can help de-escalate tension. This allows patients and families to cooperate more effectively with care instructions.

Appropriate wording:

- *Estamos haciendo todo lo posible por ayudarle.* — We are doing everything we can to help.
- *Le avisaremos tan pronto como tengamos información.* — We'll update you as soon as we have more information.
- *Gracias por su paciencia y comprensión.* — Thank you for your patience and understanding.
- *Ya viene el equipo médico. Lo van a atender de inmediato.* — The medical team is on the way. They'll take care of you right away.
- *Ya estamos cerca del hospital, tenga paciencia. Allí lo están esperando.* — We're almost at the hospital, please be patient. They're ready for you there.

## 12.3 Describing Emergency Procedures and Treatments

In emergency care, clear and compassionate communication is crucial, even when time is limited. Explaining emergency procedures, however briefly—can significantly reduce patient fear, promote cooperation, and preserve dignity during critical interventions. When interacting with Spanish-speaking patients, it is vital that providers use reassuring language that communicates both urgency and safety.

### 1 Explaining Immediate Interventions

Patients in distress benefit from brief explanations of what is being done and why. Even in a challenging environment, using calm and direct language helps create a sense of understanding and trust.

Phrases you can use to explain this to the patient

- *Vamos a administrarle oxígeno. No se retire la cánula, por favor.* — We're going to give you oxygen. Please don't remove the nasal cannula.

- *Vamos a administrarle medicamentos por vía intravenosa.* — We're going to give you IV medication.

- *Esto es para estabilizar su presión arterial / ritmo cardíaco.* — This is to stabilize your blood pressure / heart rate.

- *Debemos trasladarla a cirugía para hacer una cesárea de urgencia. El bebé está en sufrimiento, pero estamos actuando rápido para ayudarlos a ambos.* — We need to take you to the operating room for an emergency C-section. The baby is in distress, but we're acting quickly to help both of you.

- *Debemos llevarlo a una cirugía de urgencia. Su apéndice ha estallado y eso puede causar una infección grave, pero lo vamos a atender de inmediato.* — We need to take you in for emergency surgery. Your appendix has burst, and that can lead to a serious infection, but we're taking care of it right away.

- *Para pasar el catéter, debemos anestesiar la zona donde lo insertaremos. Sentirá inicialmente un pinchazo y algo de presión, pero no debería doler demasiado.* — To place the catheter, we'll need to numb the area where it will be inserted. You may feel a small pinch and some pressure at first, but it shouldn't be too painful.

### 2 Informing Patients of Diagnostic Tests

Patients should be informed about diagnostic tests, even if briefly. This fosters transparency and helps set expectations.

Phrases you can use to explain this to the patient

- *Necesitamos hacer una prueba rápida para evaluar su estado.* — We need to run a quick test to assess your condition.

- *Vamos a tomar una muestra de sangre ahora.* — We're going to take a blood sample now.

- *Esta prueba nos dirá si hay signos de infección o daño.* — This test will tell us if there are signs of infection or damage.

- *Vamos a hacerle una radiografía para saber si hay una fractura.* — We're going to take an X-ray to see if there's a fracture.

- *Le pondremos un monitor para registrar su ritmo cardíaco por unas horas.* — We'll place a monitor to record your heart rhythm for a few hours.

- *Le vamos a tomar una tomografía para buscar signos de sangrado o lesión.* — We're going to do a CT scan to look for signs of bleeding or injury.

### 3  Reassuring the Patient During Treatment

While administering treatment, continue to reassure the patient. A few calming words can help them stay still and ease their anxiety.

How to word it

- *Esto puede sentirse frío / incómodo por un momento.* — This may feel cold/uncomfortable for a moment.

- *Está en buenas manos. Estamos aquí para ayudarle.* — You're in good hands. We're here to help you.

- *Estamos monitoreando todo cuidadosamente.* — We're monitoring everything closely.

- *Todo va según lo planeado.* — Everything is going according to plan.

- *Su presión arterial está mejorando.* — Your blood pressure is improving.

- *Estamos viendo una buena respuesta al tratamiento.* — We're seeing a good response to the treatment.

- *Ya casi terminamos. Lo está haciendo muy bien.* — We're almost done. You're doing great.

- *Vamos a administrarle algo para el dolor.* — We're going to give you something for the pain.

- Describing emergency procedures, even briefly, strengthens patient-provided communication, reduces fear, and facilitates clinical cooperation. In Spanish-speaking encounters, concise and caring language can make a significant difference in how care is experienced in high-stress settings.

## 12.4 Communicating with Paramedics and Other Emergency Personnel

In emergency medicine, effective communication among healthcare professionals is as critical as clinical skill. Seamless coordination between paramedics, nurses, physicians, and other emergency personnel ensures that patients receive timely and appropriate care. When dealing with Spanish-speaking patients, bilingual communication and standardized reporting also become key elements in maintaining safety and efficiency.

## 1  Sharing Critical Information

Accurate and concise communication about a patient's status upon arrival can shape immediate decision-making. Emergency professionals must relay vital signs, observed symptoms, and prehospital treatments quickly and clearly.

Common useful expressions:

- *El paciente tiene dificultad para respirar y dolor en el pecho.* — The patient has difficulty breathing and chest pain.

- *Tiene antecedentes de asma e hipertensión.* — He/she has a history of asthma and high blood pressure.

- *Se encontraba inconsciente al llegar.* — He/she was unconscious upon arrival.

- *El paciente no responde a estímulos.* — The patient is unresponsive to stimuli.

- *Tiene una herida abierta en el abdomen.* — He/she has an open wound in the abdomen.

- *Está hipotenso, 60/30, y con pulso débil.* — He/she is hypotensive, 60/30, with a weak pulse.

- *Presenta signos de traumatismo craneoencefálico.* — He/she shows signs of head trauma.

- *La saturación de oxígeno está por debajo de 85%.* — Oxygen saturation is below 85%.

- *Tuvo una convulsión antes de llegar.* — He/she had a seizure before arrival.

- *Tiene una posible fractura expuesta en la pierna derecha.* — There's a possible open fracture in the right leg.

- *Hay sangrado activo por la nariz, los oídos y la boca.* — There is active bleeding from the nose, ears, and mouth.

- *Fue rescatado de un incendio, posible inhalación de humo.* — He/she was rescued from a fire, possible smoke inhalation.

- *Se administró epinefrina en ambulancia por sospecha de anafilaxia.* — Epinephrine was administered in the ambulance due to suspected anaphylaxis.

- *Los familiares informan que es diabético y no ha comido hoy.* — Family members report he/she is diabetic and hasn't eaten today.

- *Se aplicó desfibrilación con DEA en la ambulancia.* — Defibrillation with an AED was performed in the ambulance.

## 2  Reporting Prehospital Interventions

It is essential to document and communicate any treatment already provided during transport. This avoids duplication, prevents interactions, and supports continuity of care.

Phrases you can use to report:

- *Ya recibió una dosis de epinefrina en la ambulancia y otra en sala de Urgencias.* — He/she already received a dose of epinephrine in the ambulance and another in the ER.

- *Se administró oxígeno a 4 litros por minuto por cánula nasal.* — Oxygen was administered at 4 liters per minute, by nasal cannula.

- *Se colocó una vía intravenosa en el brazo derecho e iniciaron solución salina normal al 0.9% a 150 mL por hora para resucitación con líquidos.* — An intravenous line was established in the right arm, and 0.9% normal saline was initiated at 150 mL per hour for fluid resuscitation.

- *Se inició transfusión de glóbulos rojos empacados/empaquetados O+ en Urgencias.* — Packed red blood cell (PRBC) transfusion, type O positive, was initiated in the ER.

### 3  Coordinating Emergency Interventions

Clear direction and shared planning are critical when initiating advanced procedures. Everyone must understand their role and clinical objectives.

Phrases you can use:

- *Preparémonos para intubación.* — Let's prepare for intubation.
- *¡Iniciemos CPR / reanimación cardiopulmonar!.* — ¡Start CPR!.
- *Vamos a trasladarlo(a) directamente a la sala de trauma.* — We're taking him/her directly to the trauma bay.
- *Se activa código azul.* — Code blue activated *(Por ejemplo, empleado en contexto de paro cardiorrespiratorio / Used in case of cardiac arrest).*
- *Se activa código rojo.* — Code red activated *(En contexto de Trauma mayor que ingresa a Urgencias / Used in the context of major trauma arrival at the ER).*

Effective communication between emergency responders and clinical teams is foundational to saving lives. In fast-paced, high-stress environments, the ability to share information quickly and accurately, especially in multilingual settings can significantly impact patient outcomes.

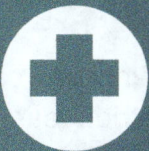

CHAPTER 13

# COMMUNICATING IN SPECIFIC SPECIALTIES

## 13.1 Obstetrics and Gynecology: Prenatal Care, Labor and Delivery

Obstetrics and gynecology involve some of the most intimate and emotionally charged conversations in healthcare. Clear, compassionate communication is essential to support pregnant patients throughout their care journey, from early prenatal visits through labor and delivery. For Spanish-speaking patients, using sensitive, respectful language fosters trust, reduces anxiety, and empowers them to participate actively in decisions concerning their health and their baby's well-being.

### 1  Initiating Prenatal Discussions

Begin every encounter with gentle, open-ended questions to establish rapport and encourage open communication about pregnancy status and early concerns.

Phrases Commonly Used:

- *¿Está embarazada o cree estarlo?* — Are you pregnant or do you think you might be?
- *¿Cuál es la fecha de su última regla (menstruación), la conoce?* — Do you know the date of your last menstrual period?
- *¿Cuántas semanas de embarazo tiene?* — How many weeks pregnant are you?
- *¿Ha tenido algún síntoma como náuseas o sangrado?* — Have you had any symptoms like nausea or bleeding?
- *¿Ha estado sintiendo al bebé?* — Have you been feeling the baby move?
- *¿Desde hace cuánto no siente al bebé moverse?* — How long has it been since you last felt the baby move?
- *¿Ha presentado algún sangrado vaginal?* — Have you had any vaginal bleeding?

## 2  Explaining Ultrasound and Routine Tests

Prenatal care often includes frequent testing to monitor the health of both mother and baby. Brief, reassuring explanations help reduce worry and encourage compliance.

Common expressions:

- *Vamos a hacer un ultrasonido para revisar al bebé y la placenta.* — We're going to do an ultrasound to check the baby and the placenta.

- *Esta prueba es para asegurarnos de que el desarrollo del bebé es normal.* — This test is to ensure the baby's development is normal.

- *También evaluaremos el nivel de líquido amniótico.* — We'll also check the amniotic fluid level.

- *Le vamos a tomar una muestra de sangre para revisar su nivel de hemoglobina.* — We'll take a blood sample to check your hemoglobin level.

- *Vamos a hacer un análisis de orina para descartar infección o presencia de proteínas.* — We're going to do a urine test to rule out infection or the presence of protein.

- *Vamos a monitorear al bebé por unos minutos para ver su frecuencia cardíaca.* — We're going to monitor the baby for a few minutes to check the heart rate.

## 3  Supporting Labor and Delivery

During labor and delivery, communication should be continuous, supportive, and calming. Prepare patients for what to expect and reassure them throughout the process.

Common expressions:

- *Durante el parto, le daremos apoyo continuo.* — During labor, we will provide continuous support.

- *Avíseme si necesita más anestesia o siente dolor.* — Let me know if you need more anesthesia or feel pain.

- *Estamos monitoreando al bebé todo el tiempo.* — We are monitoring the baby at all times.

- *Vamos a practicarle una cesárea. El bebé ha disminuido su ritmo cardíaco, lo cual indica que podría estar sufriendo.* — We're going to perform a C-section / Cesarean delivery. The baby's heart rate has dropped, which may indicate fetal distress.

- *Vamos a administrarle anestesia lumbar para que no sienta dolor durante la cesárea.* — We're going to give you spinal anesthesia so you won't feel pain during the C-section / Cesarean delivery.

## 4  Best Practices for Obstetric Communication

- Use warm, empathetic tone and non-threatening language.
- Involve partners or support persons when appropriate.
- Explain medical procedures before performing them.

- ⊙ Provide written resources in Spanish for prenatal education.
- ⊙ Normalize emotional responses and offer reassurance.

Effective communication in obstetrics and gynecology is deeply rooted in compassion, trust, and cultural sensitivity. By using clear, patient-centered Spanish-language communication, providers can ensure that patients feel respected, informed, and empowered throughout their pregnancy and delivery experience.

## 13.2 Pediatrics: Communicating with Parents and Children

Pediatric care requires a unique approach to communication that considers both the child's developmental stage and the caregiver's concerns. Effective pediatric communication in Spanish must combine medical clarity with warmth, empathy, and reassurance to help children feel safe and parents feel informed.

### 1 Engaging the Parent or Caregiver

Start by gathering essential information from the caregiver using clear and respectful questions. Parents are often anxious, so providers should create a supportive atmosphere. Please note that, culturally, grandmothers, aunts, and female cousins are part of the extended family who often play an active role in caring for children, especially during early childhood. They often provide important information about the child's medical history and background.

Sample questions for gathering information:

- ⊙ *¿Cuántos años tiene su hijo(a)?* — How old is your child?
- ⊙ *¿Ha tenido fiebre, tos o vómito? ¿Desde hace cuánto?*— Has he/she had a fever, cough, or vomiting? Since when?
- ⊙ *¿Ha cambiado su apetito o sueño?* — Has his/her appetite or sleep changed?
- ⊙ *¿Cuál es el motivo principal por el que trae a su hijo(a)?* — What is the main reason you brought your child in today?
- ⊙ *¿Ha estado en contacto con alguien enfermo recientemente?* — Has your child been in contact with anyone who is sick recently?
- ⊙ *¿Ha notado algún sarpullido, moretones o cambios en la piel?* — Have you noticed any rash, bruising, or skin changes?
- ⊙ *¿Está al día con las vacunas?* — Is your child up to date on vaccinations?
- ⊙ *¿Come y toma líquidos normalmente?* — Is your child eating and drinking normally?
- ⊙ *¿Ha perdido peso recientemente?* — Has your child lost weight recently?
- ⊙ *¿Ha tenido dificultad para respirar o se le hunden las costillas al respirar?*
- ⊙ — Has your child had trouble breathing or does the chest sink in when breathing?
- ⊙ *¿Cómo ha sido el desarrollo neurológico hasta este momento?* — How has your child's neurological development been so far?

- *¿Lo alimentó con leche materna? ¿Hasta qué edad?* — Did you breastfeed him/her? Until what age?

## 2  Speaking Directly to the Child

When appropriate, engage the child directly using simple, friendly, and informal language ("*tu*") to explain what you are doing. This helps build trust and reduces fear. Remember that children are often anxious during medical visits, so be sure to convey confidence and respect. Also, remain aware of the anxiety that both the child and their accompanying adult(s) may be experiencing.

Common useful expressions:

- *Vamos a revisar al niño(a) suavemente (si la conversación se dirige al padre).* — We're going to examine your child gently (if we are talking to the accompanying adult).
- *Vamos a revisarte suavemente (si la conversación se dirige al menor).* — We're going to examine your child gently (if we are talking directly to the child).
- *Esto no va a doler, solo quiero oír cómo están tu corazón y tus pulmones (informal porque le hablamos al niño).* — This won't hurt; I just want to listen to your heart and your lungs (informal because we are talking to the child).
- *Voy a tocar muy suavemente tu abdomen, pero avísame si te duele.* — I'm going to gently touch your tummy, but let me know if it hurts.
- *Voy a tocar muy suavemente tu cara, avísame si te duele.* — I'm going to gently touch your face, let me know if it hurts.
- *Con este aparato voy a revisar tus oídos; no te va a doler.* — I'm going to check your ears with this device; it won't hurt.
- *Abre bien grande la boca para poder revisarte.* — Open your mouth really wide so I can take a look.
- *Voy a revisar tu garganta, saca la lengua.* — I'm going to check your throat, stick out your tongue.
- *Voy a mirar tus ojos con esta luz.* — I'm going to look at your eyes with this light.
- *Vamos a pesarte y medirte para ver cuánto has crecido.* — We're going to weigh and measure you to see how much you've grown.

## 3  Reassuring the Family During the Visit

Explain procedures and findings clearly to both the parents and the child, using language appropriate to their level of understanding. Be honest about the child's condition and the proposed treatment plan, while offering reassurance and support. Ensure that both the child and their caregivers feel heard, respected, and involved in the decision-making process. This helps reduce anxiety, fosters trust, and encourages adherence to treatment.

Effective phrasing

- *Todo parece normal hasta ahora.* — Everything looks normal so far.
- *Le explicaré el tratamiento paso a paso.* — I'll explain the treatment step by step.
- *Por favor, llámenos si nota algo nuevo o preocupante.* — Please call us if you notice anything new or concerning.
- *Vamos a seguir observando y asegurarnos de que todo siga bien.* — We'll keep monitoring things to make sure everything continues to go well.
- *Entiendo que esto puede ser estresante.* — I understand this can be stressful. We're here to help.
- *Está haciendo un gran trabajo cuidando a su hijo(a).* — You're doing a great job taking care of your child.
- *Vamos a trabajar juntos para que se sienta mejor pronto.* — We'll work together to help them feel better soon.

### 4 Best Practices for Pediatric Communication

- Adapt language to both the parent and child's level of understanding.
- Use positive body language, calm tone, and gentle touch.
- Involve the parent actively in care discussions and decisions.
- Provide written discharge instructions in Spanish.
- Allow extra time for questions and emotional reassurance.

Pediatric communication is built on trust, patience, and collaboration. By using simple, kind, and clear Spanish-language communication, healthcare providers can reduce fear, improve understanding, and foster strong relationships with both children and their families throughout care.

## 13.3 Cardiology: Discussing Heart Conditions and Procedures

Cardiology discussions often carry significant emotional weight for patients, as heart conditions are commonly associated with fear and uncertainty. When communicating with Spanish-speaking patients about cardiovascular concerns, it is essential to use calm, reassuring, and precise language. Effective communication empowers patients, helps them understand their diagnosis, and promotes confidence in the recommended treatment plan.

### 1 Introducing the Diagnosis

Begin by clearly and calmly explaining the condition, using everyday language that makes it easier for the patient to understand what's happening. Speak with empathy, and allow time for the patient to absorb the news, express emotions, and ask any questions they may have.

Language examples

- *Le han diagnosticado [nombre de la condición], una enfermedad que afecta la estructura/función del corazón.* — You've been diagnosed with [name of condition], a disease that affects the heart's structure/function.

- *Su corazón no está funcionando de forma óptima, lo que significa que no está bombeando la sangre de manera eficiente al resto del cuerpo.* — Your heart is not functioning optimally, which means it is not pumping blood efficiently to the rest of your body.

- *La condición que presenta puede ser crónica, pero muchas personas viven bien con el tratamiento adecuado.* — This condition may be chronic, but many people live well with the right treatment.

- *Necesitamos hacer más pruebas para entender mejor cómo está funcionando su corazón.* — We need to do more tests to better understand how your heart is working.

- *En este momento, su condición no representa una amenaza inmediata, pero debemos actuar para evitar complicaciones.* — At this point, your condition doesn't pose an immediate threat, but we need to act to prevent complications.

- *Entiendo que esto puede ser abrumador, pero estamos aquí para acompañarle en cada paso.* — I understand this may feel overwhelming, but we are here to guide you every step of the way.

### 2 Explaining Diagnostic Tests

Clearly explain each diagnostic test, including its purpose, how it is performed, and what the patient can expect during the procedure. Use simple, non-technical language and check for understanding. Mention whether the test might cause any discomfort, if fasting or preparation is needed, whether it is outpatient or requires admission, and how long it will take to receive the results.

Speaking with empathy and honesty about the diagnosis is essential to help the patient understand their condition and feel supported throughout the process. A clear and compassionate explanation fosters trust and encourages the patient to actively participate in decisions about their treatment.

Phrases you can use to explain this to the patient

- *Vamos a hacer un electrocardiograma para evaluar el ritmo del corazón.* — We will perform an ECG to evaluate your heart rhythm.

- *Podemos realizar un ecocardiograma para observar las válvulas y el flujo de sangre.* — We may also perform an echocardiogram to examine the valves and blood flow.

- *Este examen es rápido, no duele, y nos dará información sobre la actividad eléctrica de su corazón.* — This test is quick, painless, and gives us information about your heart's electrical activity.

- *El ecocardiograma nos permite ver imágenes en movimiento del corazón para evaluar su estructura y funcionamiento.* — The echocardiogram allows us to see moving images of the heart to assess its structure and function.

- *Tal vez necesitemos una prueba de esfuerzo para ver cómo responde su corazón al ejercicio. Vamos a consultarlo con su cardiólogo* — We may need to perform a stress test to see how your heart responds to physical activity. We will consult with your cardiologist first.

- *Vamos a solicitar un monitoreo ambulatorio llamado Holter, que emplea un aparato que registra el ritmo cardíaco durante 24 horas.* — We are going to order ambulatory monitoring, called Holter monitor, which records your heart rhythm continuously.

## 3 Discussing Treatment Options

Once the diagnosis is clear, explain the available treatment options, balancing honesty with reassurance. Make sure to address any questions the patient or family may have. Describe the plan for risk management and discuss the possible outcomes, emphasizing what can be done to improve the prognosis and quality of life.

Phrases you can use to explain this to the patient

- *Es posible que necesite un cateterismo, el cual permitirá determinar si se requiere cirugía o si este procedimiento es suficiente por sí solo.* — You may need a cardiac catheterization, which will help determine whether surgery is necessary or if the procedure alone will be sufficient.

- *Le explicaremos cada paso del tratamiento antes de comenzar.* — We will explain every step of the treatment before starting.

- *El tratamiento busca estabilizar su condición y prevenir complicaciones.* — The treatment aims to stabilize your condition and prevent complications.

- *Existen diferentes opciones de tratamiento disponibles, y escogeremos la que mejor se adapte a su condición y estado general de salud.* — There are different treatment options available, and we will choose the one that best fits your condition and overall health.

- *Algunos tratamientos implican el uso de medicamentos, mientras que otros pueden requerir procedimientos o cirugía.* — Some treatments involve medication, while others may require procedures or surgery.

- *Hablemos sobre los riesgos y beneficios de cada opción para que usted pueda tomar una decisión informada.* — Let's talk about the risks and benefits of each option so you can make an informed decision.

- *Tendrá tiempo para hacer preguntas y discutir cualquier inquietud antes de continuar.* — You will have time to ask questions and discuss any concerns before we proceed.

- *El objetivo del tratamiento no es solo aliviar los síntomas, sino también mejorar la función cardíaca a largo plazo.* — The goal of the treatment is not only to relieve symptoms, but also to improve long-term heart function.

- *Los cambios en el estilo de vida así como en la dieta, el ejercicio y el manejo del estrés serán parte de su tratamiento.* — Lifestyle changes such as diet, exercise, and stress management will be part of your treatment.

### 4 Best Practices for Cardiology Communication

- Use calm, steady tone to reduce anxiety.
- Provide visual aids or written materials in Spanish.
- Encourage questions and invite family members to participate.
- Explain risks and benefits in plain language.
- Reinforce hope and the availability of effective treatments.

Cardiology conversations require both clinical precision and emotional support, just like in any other specialty.

## 13.4 Gastroenterology: Explaining Digestive Issues and Treatments

Gastroenterology involves diagnosing and managing a wide range of digestive disorders, many of which can be uncomfortable, embarrassing, or complex for patients to describe. Clear, sensitive communication in Spanish helps patients feel comfortable sharing their symptoms and better understand the procedures and treatments involved. Empowering patients with knowledge promotes cooperation and successful management of their digestive health.

### 1 Gathering Symptom Information

Start by asking simple, direct questions to help patients describe their digestive symptoms clearly. Using language encourages openness and honesty. Keep in mind that if the patient is very shy, they may have difficulty speaking freely about aspects such as the characteristics of their bowel movements, the frequency of those movements, or whether they have noticed any changes in the anal or perianal area.

Sample questions for gathering information:

- *¿Tiene dolor abdominal, distensión, gases, acidez, náuseas o sensación de llenura?* — Do you have abdominal pain, bloating, gas, heartburn, nausea, or a feeling of fullness?

- *¿Ha tenido cambios en su digestión, en la frecuencia, consistencia o aspecto de las evacuaciones, como diarrea persistente, estreñimiento o sangre en las heces?* — Have you had changes in your digestion, or in the frequency, consistency, or appearance of your bowel movements, such as persistent diarrhea, constipation, or blood in the stool?

- *¿Ha notado pérdida de peso sin una causa aparente, fatiga o sensación de evacuación incompleta? ¿Desde hace cuánto tiempo presenta estos síntomas?* — Have you noticed unexplained weight loss, fatigue, or a feeling of incomplete bowel movements? For how long have you had these symptoms?

- *¿Ha notado moco en las heces o sensación de urgencia para evacuar?* — Have you noticed mucus in your stool or a sudden urge to have a bowel movement?

- *¿Tiene fiebre, escalofríos o malestar general acompañando los síntomas digestivos?* — Have you had fever, chills, or general discomfort along with your digestive symptoms?

- *¿Ha tenido sangrado rectal o manchas de sangre en el papel higiénico?* — Have you had rectal bleeding or noticed blood on the toilet paper?

- *¿Ha notado bultos dolorosos, ardor o picazón alrededor del ano, especialmente después de evacuar?* — Have you noticed painful lumps, burning, or itching around the anus, especially after a bowel movement?

## 2 Explaining Diagnostic Procedures

Many gastrointestinal conditions require procedures such as endoscopy, blood test and stool analysis to obtain an accurate diagnosis. Briefly explaining these tests can help reduce patient anxiety or reluctance. It is also important to explain that although endoscopic procedures may be uncomfortable, they can be performed under mild sedation to minimize discomfort. Therefore, it is advisable for a responsible adult to accompany the patient on the day of the procedure, especially to provide support afterward.

Common useful expressions:

- *Es necesario hacer una endoscopia para observar el interior del sistema digestivo.* — An endoscopy may be needed to examine the digestive tract.

- *Este procedimiento nos ayudará a identificar la causa de sus síntomas.* — This procedure will help us identify the cause of your symptoms.

- *Necesita una gastroscopia para revisar especialmente su estómago y excluir la presencia de alguna lesión.* — You need a gastroscopy to closely examine your stomach and rule out any lesions.

- *Necesita una colonoscopia para revisar la presencia de pólipos o de alguna otra lesión en su colon.* — You need a colonoscopy to check for polyps or any other lesions in your colon.

- *Necesito revisar su zonas anal y perianal buscando algún tipo de lesión.* — I need to examine your anal and perianal area to look for any type of lesion.

## 3 Presenting Treatment Options

Gastrointestinal care often involves a combination of lifestyle adjustments, dietary changes, and medications. Clear explanations help patients commit to long-term management. In many cases, additional procedures such as endoscopy or stool analysis are also required to accurately diagnose and monitor the condition. Together, these measures are essential for effectively controlling the disease and its symptoms, improving quality of life, and preventing complications.

Common useful expressions:

- *Recomendamos cambios en la dieta y medicamentos específicos para su tratamiento.* — We recommend dietary changes and specific medications.

- *Un factor clave es que usted evite alimentos que irriten el sistema digestivo, como los picantes, los condimentos fuertes, los fritos y los productos lácteos si causan molestias.* — A major factor is that you avoid foods that irritate the digestive system, such as spicy foods, strong seasonings, fried foods, and dairy products if they cause discomfort.

- *Algunos pacientes responden bien solo con cambios en la dieta, mientras que otros necesitan medicamentos.* — Some patients respond well to diet alone, while others may require medications.

- *Si los síntomas no mejoran con estas medidas, consideraremos pruebas adicionales o tratamientos más avanzados.* — If symptoms do not improve with these measures, we will consider additional tests or more advanced treatments.

- *Cada opción tiene posibles beneficios y riesgos; hablaremos sobre cada uno para que pueda tomar una decisión informada.* — Each option has potential benefits and risks; we'll discuss them so you can make an informed decision.

- *En algunos casos, también puede estar indicada la suplementación con probióticos o fibra, según la causa.* — In some cases, supplementation with probiotics or fiber may also be indicated, depending on the underlying cause.

## 4 Best Practices for Gastroenterology Communication

- Create a comfortable environment to discuss sensitive symptoms.
- Use clear language to describe procedures and what to expect.
- Provide written dietary guidelines in Spanish.
- Encourage patients to report any new or worsening symptoms.
- Reinforce that many digestive issues are manageable with proper care.

Gastroenterology communication, like any other specialty, requires both clinical clarity and emotional sensitivity. Spanish-speaking patients benefit greatly from clear, supportive explanations that help them understand their condition and take an active role in managing their digestive health.

### Caso Clínico

*Este caso clínico resalta la importancia de una comunicación efectiva en el contexto de los cuidados paliativos, donde un enfoque interdisciplinario, claro y compasivo es esencial para brindar una atención integral al paciente y su familia. Una comunicación adecuada no solo permite comprender el proceso clínico y aliviar el sufrimiento, sino que también mejora el acceso a la información necesaria para que la familia se involucre activamente en el cuidado, favoreciendo la toma de decisiones compartida y respetando los valores y deseos del paciente.*

## Presentación del caso

El paciente es el señor Pérez, un hombre de 70 años con diagnóstico de cáncer de próstata avanzado, en etapa terminal. Ha sido remitido al equipo de cuidados paliativos para recibir atención en casa que le ayude a controlar el dolor y aliviar los síntomas.

## Equipo de cuidados paliativos

- Oncólogo: Dr. García
- Especialista en cuidados paliativos / Paliativista: Dra. Martínez
- Enfermera: Enfermera López
- Psicóloga: Dra. González
- Trabajador Social: Señor Ramírez

## Reunión clínica conjunta: oncólogo, paliativista y paciente

*Dr. García (oncólogo):* Señor Pérez, entiendo que estos últimos días han sido especialmente difíciles. Hemos llegado a una etapa en la que el enfoque principal debe ser su bienestar y comodidad. Por eso quisimos reunirnos con el equipo médico de cuidados paliativos.

*Dra. Martínez (médica paliativista):* Señor Pérez, gracias por estar con nosotros hoy. Estamos aquí con el Dr. García, su oncólogo, para conversar juntos sobre cómo se ha sentido últimamente y revisar las opciones para aliviar su malestar.

*Sr. Pérez (paciente):* Gracias, doctora. La verdad me siento muy agotado... el dolor no me deja dormir y ya casi no tengo fuerzas para levantarme. Además, todo lo que como me cae mal y tengo náuseas y vómitos frecuentes con casi todas mis comidas. Me siento emocionalmente afectado: tengo ansiedad y me siento deprimido con frecuencia.

*Dr. García:* Señor Pérez, entiendo que estos últimos días han sido especialmente difíciles. Hemos llegado a una etapa en la que el enfoque principal debe ser su bienestar y comodidad. Comprendo, señor Pérez. Todos estos síntomas son esperables en esta etapa de la enfermedad, lo ayudaremos a disminuir ese malestar. Podemos trabajar juntos para reducir esa carga.

*Dra. Martínez:* Exactamente. Vamos a hacer algunos ajustes para controlar mejor el dolor, y también revisaremos los medicamentos para manejar las náuseas y mejorar su tolerancia alimentaria. Además, me gustaría que nuestra psicóloga y el trabajador social lo acompañaran para brindarle apoyo emocional a usted y a su familia.

*Sr. Pérez:* Me parece bien. Me da tranquilidad saber que están todos pendientes y que no solo se enfocan en la enfermedad, sino también en cómo me siento y cómo está mi familia. Me preocupa ser una carga para mi esposa.

*Dr. García:* Esa es justamente la idea, señor Pérez. Su bienestar es nuestra prioridad.

*Dra. Martínez: Además, podemos coordinar su atención en casa. Nos aseguraremos de que usted y su esposa reciban todo el apoyo necesario. ¿Le parece bien si empezamos hoy con unos ajustes y nos volvemos a ver en unos días para evaluar cómo se siente?*

*Sr. Pérez: Sí, doctora.* Me siento más tranquilo al saber que cuento con su apoyo.

## Reunión equipo de cuidados paliativos

*Dr. García (oncólogo): Dra. Martínez, ¿cómo está respondiendo el señor Pérez al tratamiento para el dolor y sus otras molestias?*

*Dra. Martínez (paliativista): Está mejorando lentamente. Hemos hecho algunos ajustes en la medicación para controlar mejor el dolor, y también estamos implementando estrategias para manejar la fatiga y la ansiedad. Además, modificamos su tratamiento para las náuseas y los vómitos, dando recomendaciones alimentarias; hasta ahora ha tenido una respuesta positiva, con menos episodios y mejor tolerancia a los alimentos.*

*Enfermera López: He notado que el señor Pérez tiene dificultades para dormir. ¿Podemos considerar alguna intervención adicional para ayudarlo?*

*Dra. Martínez: Sí, definitivamente. Vamos a explorar opciones farmacológicas suaves y también algunas medidas no farmacológicas para mejorar su descanso.*

*Dra. González (psicóloga): He conversado con el señor Pérez y expresa sentimientos persistentes de ansiedad y tristeza, asociados con su pérdida de funcionalidad y dependencia. Estoy trabajando con él en técnicas de manejo emocional y en la validación de su experiencia para disminuir su angustia. Si no responde en forma adecuada propongo intervenir con medicamentos.*

*Señor Ramírez (trabajador social): La esposa del señor Pérez me manifestó que se siente abrumada y teme no poder cuidar de él adecuadamente en casa. Estoy buscando apoyo para que puedan recibir ayuda en casa, y orientando a su esposa para que no se sienta sola en este proceso.*

## Plan de cuidados

- ⊙ *Manejo del dolor: Ajustar la medicación de forma continua según la intensidad del dolor y la respuesta del paciente, priorizando la comodidad.*

- ⊙ *Manejo de síntomas gastrointestinales: Optimizar el tratamiento de las náuseas y vómitos para mejorar la tolerancia alimentaria y reducir el malestar.*

- ⊙ *Apoyo emocional y psicológico: Brindar intervención psicológica para abordar la ansiedad, la depresión y el impacto emocional del proceso de enfermedad, tanto para el paciente como para su familia.*

- ⊙ *Mejorar el descanso: Implementar estrategias farmacológicas y no farmacológicas para tratar el insomnio y mejorar la calidad del sueño.*

- *Apoyo psicosocial: Evaluar las necesidades sociales del paciente y su familia, incluyendo aspectos económicos, de cuidado y red de apoyo, con participación del trabajador social.*

- *Cuidados en el hogar: Coordinar con el equipo de cuidados paliativos para garantizar atención continua en el domicilio, incluyendo visitas médicas, de enfermería y acompañamiento psicosocial.*

## Clinical Case (English Version)

This clinical case highlights the importance of effective communication in the context of palliative care, where a clear, compassionate, and interdisciplinary approach is essential to provide comprehensive support to both the patient and their family. Proper communication not only helps in understanding the clinical process and alleviating suffering, but also improves access to the information needed for the family to actively participate in the patient's care, supporting shared decision-making and respecting the patient's values and wishes.

### Case Presentation

The patient is Mr. Pérez, a 70-year-old man diagnosed with advanced, terminal-stage prostate cancer. He has been referred to the palliative care team to help manage his pain and other symptoms at home.

### Palliative Care Team

- Oncologist: Dr. García
- Palliative Care Specialist: Dr. Martínez
- Nurse: Nurse López
- Psychologist: Dr. González
- Social Worker: Mr. Ramírez

### Joint Clinical Meeting: Oncologist, Palliative Care Specialist, and Patient

Dr. García (Oncologist): Mr. Pérez, I understand these past few days have been especially difficult. We've reached a point where our main focus should be your comfort and well-being. That's why we've invited the palliative care team to join us.

Dr. Martínez (Palliative Care Physician): Mr. Pérez, thank you for being with us today. Dr. García and I are here to talk together about how you've been feeling and to review some options to help ease your discomfort.

Mr. Pérez (Patient): Thank you, doctor. Honestly, I feel extremely tired... the pain keeps me from sleeping, and I barely have the strength to get out of bed. Also, everything I eat upsets my stomach—I have frequent nausea and vomiting with almost every meal. I feel emotionally affected, often anxious, and quite depressed.

Dr. García: I hear you, Mr. Pérez. All of these symptoms are expected at this stage of illness. We're here to help you feel more comfortable. We'll work together to ease that burden.

Dr. Martínez: Exactly. We'll make some adjustments to help control the pain better, and also review the medications that might ease your nausea and improve your ability to tolerate food. In addition, I'd like our psychologist and social worker to support you and your family emotionally during this time.

Mr. Pérez: That sounds good. It reassures me to know that you're all paying attention, not just to the disease, but also to how I feel and how my family is coping. I worry about being a burden to my wife.

Dr. García: That's exactly the idea, Mr. Pérez. Your well-being is our priority.

Dr. Martínez: We can also coordinate your care at home. We'll make sure you and your wife feel supported and have everything you need at home. Does it sound good to start with some adjustments today and meet again in a few days to see how you're feeling?

Mr. Pérez: Yes, doctor. I feel more at ease knowing I have your support.

Interdisciplinary Palliative Care Team Meeting

Dr. García (Oncologist): Dr. Martínez, how is Mr. Pérez responding to the treatment for his pain and other symptoms?

Dr. Martínez (Palliative Care Specialist): He's improving gradually. We've made some adjustments to his medication to better control the pain, and we're also implementing strategies to manage fatigue and anxiety. Additionally, we modified his treatment for nausea and vomiting and provided dietary recommendations. So far, he's had a positive response, with fewer episodes and better food tolerance.

Nurse López: I've noticed that Mr. Pérez is having trouble sleeping. Should we consider any additional interventions to help with that?

Dr. Martínez: Yes, definitely. We'll explore some gentle pharmacological options as well as non-pharmacological strategies to improve his rest.

Dr. González (Psychologist): I've spoken with Mr. Pérez, and he reports persistent feelings of anxiety and sadness related to his loss of functionality and growing dependence. I'm working with him on emotional coping techniques and validating his experience to reduce distress. If he doesn't respond adequately, I would suggest considering medication.

Mr. Ramírez (Social Worker): Mr. Pérez's wife shared with me that she feels overwhelmed and is afraid she won't be able to care for him properly at home. I'm arranging for support at home and guiding her so she doesn't feel alone in this process.

<u>Care Plan</u>

- Pain management: Continuously adjust medication based on pain intensity and patient response, prioritizing comfort.

- Gastrointestinal symptom control: Optimize treatment for nausea and vomiting to improve food tolerance and reduce discomfort.

- Emotional and psychological support: Provide psychological intervention to address anxiety, depression, and emotional impact of the illness, both for the patient and family.

- Improving sleep: Implement both pharmacologic and non-pharmacologic strategies to manage insomnia and enhance sleep quality.

- Psychosocial support: Assess social needs of the patient and family, including financial, caregiving, and support network aspects, with the involvement of the social worker.

- Home-based care: Coordinate with the palliative care team to ensure continuous care at home, including medical visits, nursing care, and psychosocial support.

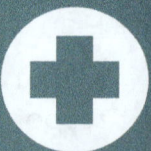

CHAPTER 14

# PROVIDING HEALTH EDUCATION MATERIALS IN SPANISH

## 14.1 Understanding Cultural Considerations in Health Education

Effective health education is not only about translating words, but also about delivering information in a way that respects and reflects the cultural values, beliefs, and traditions of the patient population. For Spanish-speaking communities, cultural considerations are deeply intertwined with health decision-making, communication styles, and family dynamics.

Healthcare providers must develop culturally appropriate materials that foster trust, promote understanding, and support informed decision-making.

### 1  Acknowledging Family-Centered Decision-Making

In many Hispanic and Latino cultures, family plays a vital role in health decisions. When appropriate, including family members in discussions and care planning helps create a collaborative environment and fosters trust, while also respecting their influence and cultural values. This consideration is equally important when caring for children, as extended and close family members may play a key role in the child's care.

Suggested phrases for typical patient encounters:

- *Algunos pacientes valoran la opinión de la familia en decisiones médicas. Podemos programar una reunión familiar si usted lo desea* — Some patients value family input in medical decisions. We can schedule a family meeting if you'd like

- *¿Quiere que un miembro de su familia participe en esta conversación?* — Would you like a family member to join this conversation?

- *¿Hay alguien en su familia a quien deberíamos mantener informado?* — Is there someone in your family we should keep informed?

- *Comprendemos que la familia puede ser un apoyo emocional importante.* — We understand that family can be an important source of emotional support.

- *¿Quién suele tomar las decisiones médicas en su familia? (Esta pregunta es especialmente relevante en casos donde el paciente está inconsciente, tiene capacidad de decisión disminuida o ausente, o se trata de un menor de edad. Nos ayuda a identificar si existe un representante legal designado para la toma de decisiones.)* — Who usually makes medical decisions in your family? (This is particularly important when the patient is unconscious, has diminished or absent decision-making capacity, or is a minor. It helps us determine if there is a legally designated decision-maker.)

- *Es importante para nosotros respetar sus creencias y dinámicas familiares.* — It's important for us to respect your family beliefs and dynamics.

- *¿Le gustaría que su familia estuviera presente durante esta explicación?* — Would you like your family to be present during this explanation?

- *Podemos brindar información a su familia si usted lo autoriza.* — We can share information with your family if you authorize us to do so.

- *Tenga en cuenta que el tono corporal y el contacto visual pueden tener significados distintos entre culturas. Siempre busque señales de incomodidad en su interlocutor.* — Be aware that body language and eye contact can have different meanings across cultures. Always watch for signs of discomfort in the person you're speaking with.

## 2   Using Respectful and Appropriate Language

Health education in printed or electronic materials, as well as in talks, should be delivered in a tone that is respectful, compassionate, and free of jargon. Culturally appropriate language acknowledges and respects patient values while conveying clear and accurate medical information. Always provide clear instructions and explain the process for requesting additional information.

Key Considerations:

- *Preste atención al empleo de un lenguaje respetuoso y apropiado.* — Pay attention to use respectful and community-appropriate language.

- *Evite términos médicos complicados. Siempre dé explicaciones en los términos más sencillos que sea posible y adecuado a la situación.* — Let's avoid complicated medical terms; always explain using simple words.

- *Evite ser condescendiente* — Avoid being condescending.

- *Adapte el material educativo al nivel cultural y educativo de su comunidad.* — Adapt educational materials to the patient's cultural and educational background.

- *Considere que hay creencias culturales o religiosas que puedan influir en la aceptación de la información médica.* — Consider whether cultural or religious beliefs may affect how the medical information is received.

- *No asuma que todos los miembros de una misma comunidad piensan igual.* — Do not assume all members of a cultural group think or believe the same.

### 3  Adapting Materials to the Community's Needs

Health education should reflect not only language, but also community-specific beliefs about health, illness, and healing. Materials should address common concerns, emphasize prevention, and promote healthy habits in relatable ways.

Important Points When Communicating Health Information Across Cultures:

- Include culturally relevant examples and visuals.
- Recognize and validate traditional health practices when safe.
- Provide information about how to navigate the healthcare system.
- Encourage open dialogue and shared decision-making.
- Be aware of language barriers and always offer interpreter services if needed.
- Avoid assumptions based on ethnicity, clothing, or accent.
- Clarify consent processes in culturally sensitive ways.
- Keep the information you share up to date.

### 4  Best Practices for Culturally Competent Health Education

- Involve bilingual and bicultural staff in developing materials.
- Pilot test materials with members of the target community.
- Offer both written and verbal explanations.
- Be sensitive to religious, spiritual, and cultural beliefs.
- Emphasize respect, empathy, and patient empowerment.

Culturally responsive health education in Spanish helps bridge gaps in understanding and builds stronger relationships between healthcare providers and patients. When providers respect cultural values while sharing accurate information, they don't just give care—they build trust. This connection encourages healthier choices and better health outcomes for diverse communities.

## 14.2 Adapting English Materials into Clear and Culturally Sensitive Spanish

Creating effective Spanish-language health education materials involves more than simple translation. True adaptation requires an understanding of both language and culture, ensuring that information is not only accurate but also relevant, respectful, and easily understood by Spanish-speaking patients. When properly adapted, these materials foster trust, promote better health outcomes, and empower patients to engage more fully in their care.

## 1 Going Beyond Word-for-Word Translation

Direct translations often fail to convey the intended meaning, especially when cultural context or healthcare systems differ. Professional translations should adapt the content while maintaining its clinical integrity. Be aware that literal translations can lead to confusion or misunderstandings.

Some good practices are:

- *Lo adecuado es no solo traducir palabra por palabra, sino también tener en cuenta el contexto.* — It's best not to translate word for word, but to take the context into account.

- *El significado debe ser claro y respetuoso para el paciente.* — The meaning must be clear and respectful for the patient.

- *Asegúrese de que la traducción mantenga la intención y el tono del mensaje* original. — Make sure the translation preserves the intent and tone of the original message.

- *Considere emplear modismos o expresiones locales que podrían no tener una equivalencia directa, si la situación lo amerita.* — Consider using local idioms or expressions that may not have a direct equivalent, if the situation calls for it.

- *Siempre revise y, si es posible, pruebe el material con miembros de la comunidad a la que está dirigido.* — Always review and, if possible, test the material with members of the target community.

- *Verifique con personal de salud de habla española o latinos, que el contenido sea claro y efectivo.* — Check with Spanish-speaking or Latino healthcare staff to ensure the content is clear and effective.

## 2 Using Relevant Examples and Common Phrases

Culturally adapted materials include familiar expressions, relatable examples, and culturally appropriate analogies. This ensures that patients can connect with the information and apply it to their daily lives.

Suggested Methodology:

- *Use ejemplos relevantes y frases comunes en español.* — Use relevant examples and common Spanish phrases.

- *Incluya referencias culturales que sean significativas para la comunidad.* — Include cultural references that are meaningful to the community.

## 3 Ensuring Accuracy and Cultural Sensitivity

It's essential to balance medical accuracy with cultural sensitivity. Avoid idioms, slang, or humor that may not translate well or could cause offense. Use them only if you're certain that they enhance clarity and effectiveness.

Key points:

- ⊙ Avoid complex medical jargon unless explained.
- ⊙ Use simple, patient-friendly language.
- ⊙ Consult with bilingual, bicultural healthcare professionals.
- ⊙ Test materials with native Spanish speakers.
- ⊙ Ensure cultural relevance and appropriateness of examples or images.
- ⊙ Be aware of regional language differences among Spanish-speaking communities.
- ⊙ Use plain-language design principles (short sentences, clear headings, visual aids).

**4** **Best Practices for Adapting Educational Materials**

- ⊙ Collaborate with professional medical translators.
- ⊙ Involve community members in reviewing drafts.
- ⊙ Ensure consistency in terminology across materials.
- ⊙ Offer materials in both printed and electronic formats when possible.
- ⊙ Follow CLAS Standards (ensure equity, respect, and language access)

Properly adapted health education materials reflect both linguistic and cultural fluency. By prioritizing clarity, relevance, and respect, healthcare providers can build trust with Spanish-speaking patients, ensuring that health education truly informs and empowers diverse populations.

## 14.3 Explaining Complex Medical Information in Lay Terms

One of the most important skills in healthcare communication is the ability to translate complex medical concepts into language that patients can easily understand. Spanish-speaking patients, like all patients, benefit from clear, simplified explanations that remove medical jargon while maintaining accuracy. Simplifying medical information not only improves comprehension but also empowers patients to actively participate in their care and make informed decisions.

**1** **Simplifying Medical Terms**

Use plain language whenever possible. Replace technical terms with words that are more familiar to patients while still conveying the correct meaning.

# Plain Language Alternatives for Medical Terms

| Término médico (español) | Medical Term (English) | Lenguaje sencillo (español) |
| --- | --- | --- |
| Hipertensión | high blood pressure | Presión alta |
| Hipoglucemia | Hypoglycemia | Azúcar baja en la sangre |
| Hiperglucemia | Hyperglycemia | Azúcar alta en la sangre |
| Colesterol elevado | Hypercholesterolemia | Colesterol alto |
| Enfermedad cardiovascular | Cardiovascular disease | Enfermedad del corazón o del sistema circulatorio |
| Infarto agudo de miocardio | Acute myocardial infarction (AMI) | Ataque al corazón |
| Accidente cerebrovascular | Cerebrovascular accident (CVA) / Stroke | Derrame cerebral |
| Disnea | Dyspnea | Dificultad para respirar / Falta de aire |
| Dolor torácico | Chest pain | Dolor en el pecho |
| Náusea | Nausea | Ganas de vomitar |
| Cefalea | Headache | Dolor de cabeza |
| Astenia / Fatiga | Asthenia / Fatigue | Cansancio extremo |
| Edema | Edema | Hinchazón |
| Antiinflamatorios | Anti-inflammatory drugs | Medicamentos para la inflamación |
| Hemorragia | Hemorrhage | Sangrado |
| Infección urinaria | Urinary tract infection (UTI) | Infección en la orina |
| Lesión | Injury / Lesion | Herida |
| Efectos secundarios | Side effects | Reacciones no deseadas del medicamento |
| Hematoma | Hematoma | Morado / Moretón / Cardenal |

## 2   Avoiding Medical Jargon

Medical terminology often includes complex words that may not translate well or may confuse patients. Eliminate or explain unfamiliar words, especially those related to anatomy, procedures, or pharmacology.

Key points:

- *Evite jergas médicas que puedan causar confusión.* — Avoid medical jargon that may cause confusion.

- *Si necesita usar un término médico, explíquelo de inmediato en palabras sencillas.* — If you need to use a medical term, explain it immediately in simple words.

## 3   Using Visuals and Analogies

Visual aids and familiar comparisons can help explain complicated processes. This makes abstract ideas more relatable and memorable for patients.

Helpful strategies include:

- *Use diagramas o imágenes para explicar anatomía o procedimientos.* —Use diagrams or images to explain anatomy or procedures.

- *Apoye con ayudas visuales como: ilustraciones, infografías, videos o animaciones simples.* — Support with visual aids such as illustrations, infographics, short videos, or simple animations.

- *Utilice analogías cotidianas (ej. vasos sanguíneos = tuberías de agua) para facilitar la comprensión.* — Use everyday analogies (e.g., blood vessels = water pipes) to aid understanding.

- *Explique porciones o nutrición con alimentos familiares (ej. proteína = tamaño de una baraja).* — Use familiar foods to explain nutrition (e.g., protein = size of a deck of cards).

- *Relacione la toma de medicamentos con rutinas diarias (ej. desayuno, antes de dormir).* — Relate medication schedules to daily routines (e.g., breakfast, bedtime).

- *Use gestos, tono de voz y expresiones para reforzar el mensaje.* — Use gestures, tone of voice, and facial expressions to reinforce meaning.

- *Repita los puntos clave y verifique comprensión con "enséñeme lo que entendió".* —Repeat key points and check understanding with "teach-back" methods.

- *Evite conceptos abstractos: use ejemplos concretos y visibles.* — Avoid abstract concepts: use clear, concrete examples.

## 4   Best Practices for Simplifying Medical Information

- Avoid acronyms and abbreviations.
- Speak slowly and clearly.
- Pause frequently to check understanding.

- Use the teach-back method to confirm comprehension.
- Provide written materials in plain Spanish for reinforcement.

Simplifying medical language is a vital component of patient-centered care. By breaking down complex concepts into clear, relatable Spanish, healthcare professionals can help patients feel confident, respected, and fully involved in their health decisions, leading to better outcomes and stronger provider-patient relationships.

## 14.4 Utilizing Other Educational Resources

Visual aids and educational resources can be powerful tools to help patients better understand their care. For Spanish-speaking patients, well-designed visuals, videos, and culturally appropriate materials can bridge communication gaps, simplify complex information, and empower patients to take a more active role in managing their health.

### 1 The Power of Visual Learning

Visuals help explain difficult concepts in a clear, memorable way. They reduce reliance on written text and allow patients to better visualize anatomy, procedures, treatment plans, and lifestyle changes.

Useful approaches include:

- *Use diagramas, dibujos y folletos ilustrativos.* — Use diagrams, drawings, and illustrated brochures.
- *Los diagramas pueden mostrar claramente dónde está el problema en el cuerpo.* — Diagrams can clearly show where the problem is in the body.
- *Utilice infografías digitales para explicar condiciones comunes.* — Use digital infographics to explain common conditions.
- *Use aplicaciones o programas con modelos 3D del cuerpo humano.* — Use apps or programs with 3D models of the human body.

### 2 Leveraging Video and Multimedia Tools

Spanish-language videos can reinforce verbal education, demonstrate procedures, and provide patients with accessible, repeatable instructions that they can watch at home.

The Power of Video in Health Education:

- *Los videos en español pueden ser herramientas educativas efectivas.* — Spanish-language videos can be effective educational tools.
- *Los videos pueden enseñar técnicas de cuidado personal o ejercicios de rehabilitación.* — Videos can teach self-care techniques or rehabilitation exercises.

### 3  Adapting Materials to Literacy Levels

Educational resources should be designed with consideration for the wide range of literacy and education levels within Spanish-speaking populations. Use simple language, large print, and culturally relevant imagery.

Effective Strategies:

- ◉ Use pictures to support every major point.
- ◉ Keep text short and in plain Spanish.
- ◉ Include clear instructions with step-by-step visuals.
- ◉ Review materials with patients to ensure understanding.

### 4  Best Practices for Using Educational Resources

- ◉ Involve patients actively in reviewing the materials.
- ◉ Use bilingual or bicultural staff to develop and present resources.
- ◉ Regularly update materials to ensure medical accuracy.
- ◉ Encourage patients to share materials with family members.
- ◉ Evaluate patient comprehension through teaching or discussion.

Incorporating visual aids and educational resources into patient care can transform complex medical information into clear, actionable guidance.

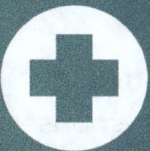

## CHAPTER 15

# CONDUCTING PATIENT COUNSELING AND MOTIVATIONAL INTERVIEWING

## 15.1 Building Trust and Empathy in Counseling Sessions

Patient counseling and motivational interviewing are most effective when grounded in trust, empathy, and open communication. These techniques are vital for guiding Spanish-speaking patients through complex decisions, behavioral changes, or emotional challenges. By fostering a safe space where patients feel heard and respected, healthcare professionals can better support long-term engagement and positive health outcomes.

### 1 Communicating with Respect and Compassion

Begin each counseling session by expressing empathy and assuring the patient that they are in a safe and judgment-free environment. Use simple, compassionate Spanish that invites openness.

Phrases to Foster Trust and Emotional Safety:

- *Mi objetivo con esta charla es escucharle sin juzgarle y brindarle toda mi ayuda.* — My goal in this conversation is to listen to you without judgment and offer you my full support.

- *Mi compromiso es con su bienestar y su salud.* — My commitment is to your well-being and health.

- *Lo que me diga y lo que hablemos es confidencial.* — What you tell me and what we discuss is confidential.

- *Estoy aquí para acompañarle y brindarle un espacio seguro donde pueda expresar sus dudas y temores.* — I'm here to support you and provide a safe space where you can express your doubts and fears.

- *Recuerde que puede contar con un equipo de apoyo psicosocial que lo oriente y apoye.* — Remember that you can count on a psychosocial support team to guide and assist you.

**2** **Encouraging Expression of Concerns**

Invite the patient to share their thoughts, fears, or questions. Active listening and thoughtful responses help uncover underlying issues that may affect compliance or emotional well-being.

Some examples of ways to communicate with respect and care:

- *Cuénteme lo que le preocupa. Esa información será tratada en forma confidencial.* — Tell me what's worrying you. That information will be kept confidential.

- *¿Qué le gustaría cambiar o mejorar en su salud?* — What would you like to change or improve about your health?

- *No hay preguntas equivocadas ni preocupaciones pequeñas.* — There are no wrong questions or small concerns.

- *Lo que usted siente es válido, y esta conversación es para atender esas inquietudes.* — What you're feeling is valid, and this conversation is meant to address those concerns.

- *Abrirse sin temor está bien.* — It's okay to open up.

- *Está bien expresarse libremente.* — It's okay to express yourself freely.

**3** **Demonstrating Active Listening and Validation**

Nonverbal cues—such as eye contact, facial expressions, posture, and tone of voice—play a crucial role in communication. Paying attention to both the provider's and the patient's nonverbal signals fosters mutual understanding. When combined with reflective statements and affirmations, these behaviors demonstrate that the provider is truly listening, helping to build rapport and strengthen the therapeutic relationship.

Strategies that can be used:

- *Evite interrumpir al paciente, especialmente si no está de acuerdo. La corrección debe hacerse con empatía y cordialidad, manteniendo siempre el rumbo clínico de la consulta.* — Avoid interrupting the patient, especially if you disagree. Corrections should be made with empathy and kindness, while maintaining clinical direction during the consultation.

- *Mantenga contacto visual y asienta con la cabeza para mostrar interés.* — Maintain eye contact and nod to show engagement.

- *Refleje lo que dice el paciente utilizando sus propias palabras.* — Reflect what the patient says using their words.

- *Valide las emociones con frases como: "Entiendo que eso debe ser difícil."* — Validate emotions with phrases like: "I understand that must be difficult."

- *Use gestos y expresiones mínimas (como "sí", "entiendo", o movimientos de cabeza) para animar al paciente a continuar.* — Use small verbal or physical cues (like "yes," "I see," or head nods) to encourage the patient to keep sharing.

- *Resuma o parafrasee lo que ha dicho el paciente para mostrar comprensión y dar oportunidad de corregir o profundizar.* — Summarize or paraphrase what the patient said to show understanding and allow for clarification or elaboration.

- *Dé espacios para que el paciente piense sobre lo que se le ha dicho.* — Give the patient time to reflect on what has been said.

### 4  Best Practices for Building Trust in Counseling

- Begin sessions with a warm, respectful tone.
- Set clear expectations about confidentiality.
- Encourage small steps toward change.
- Use the patient's preferred name and pronouns.
- Recognize and affirm patient strengths and efforts.

Trust and empathy are not optional; they are essential for effective counseling and motivational interviewing. By creating a supportive, respectful environment and using culturally sensitive Spanish-language communication, providers can help patients feel seen, understood, and motivated to engage in their care.

## 15.2 Addressing Patient Fears and Misconceptions

Fear and misinformation often prevent patients from fully engaging in treatment or following medical advice. When working with Spanish-speaking patients, healthcare providers must gently address these concerns with patience, empathy, and cultural sensitivity. By clarifying misunderstandings and validating emotions, providers help build trust and promote healthier, better-informed decisions.

### 1  Normalizing Fear and Uncertainty

Patients may feel anxious or ashamed about expressing their fears. Start by validating their emotions and reassuring them that their concerns are common and understandable.

Sample expressions:

- *Es normal tener dudas o miedo.* — It's normal to have doubts or fears.
- *Muchas personas sienten lo mismo al enfrentar un diagnóstico nuevo.* — Many people feel the same when facing a new diagnosis.

### 2  Exploring Patient Beliefs and Information Sources

Encourage patients to share what they've heard or believe about their condition or treatment. This helps identify any myths or misinformation that need to be addressed.

Example Phrases:

- *¿Qué conoce sobre esta enfermedad?* — What do you know about this condition?

- *¿Conoce o ha escuchado (oído) sobre este medicamento, terapia o examen?* — Do you know about or have you heard of this medication, therapy, or test?

- *Me gustaría saber cuáles son sus preocupaciones específicas.* — I would like to know what your specific concerns are.

- *¿Ha buscado información sobre este tema en Internet, ha hablado con alguien, como familiares, amigos, profesionales de salud, o incluso ha consultado con inteligencia artificial?* — Have you looked up information about this topic online, talked to anyone, such as family, friends, healthcare professionals, or even consulted with artificial intelligence?

### 3 Explaining Treatment Safety and Benefits

Use simple, reassuring language to explain why the recommended treatment is both safe and beneficial, while remaining open to patient questions.

Phrasing options

- *Permítame explicarle por qué este tratamiento es seguro y necesario.* — Let me explain why this treatment is safe and necessary.

- *Permítame explicarle los beneficios y riesgos de este tratamiento.* — Let me explain the benefits and risks of this treatment.

**Nota**: *Muchos pacientes valoran recibir información clara y honesta sobre los posibles riesgos, complicaciones y la evolución esperada de su enfermedad. Cuando es pertinente, puede ser útil proporcionar datos numéricos —como probabilidades o porcentajes— para apoyar la comprensión y facilitar la toma de decisiones informadas. Sin embargo, estas cifras deben explicarse en un lenguaje sencillo y adaptarse al nivel de alfabetización en salud del paciente. También es importante ser sensible: asegúrese de transmitir la información con un tono sereno y tranquilizador, resaltando las medidas tomadas para reducir los riesgos y aumentar la seguridad del tratamiento.* — **Note**: Many patients appreciate receiving clear, honest information about the potential risks, complications, and expected course of their condition. When appropriate, it can be helpful to provide numerical data—such as probabilities or percentages—to support understanding and informed decision-making. However, these figures should be explained in plain language and tailored to the patient's level of health literacy. Sensitivity is also important: ensure that the information is shared in a calm, reassuring tone, emphasizing the measures taken to reduce risks and enhance treatment safety.

### 4 Best Practices for Addressing Fears and Misconceptions

- Listen carefully without judgment.

- Ask open-ended questions to uncover hidden concerns.

- Avoid dismissive language; acknowledge all emotions.
- Provide culturally appropriate education and resources.
- Normalize fears to reduce stigma.
- Reassure the patient about your role in supporting their decision-making process
- Use teach-back to verify understanding and correct misinformation.

Addressing patient fears and misconceptions is a delicate but crucial part of counseling and motivational interviewing. By creating a safe, respectful environment where Spanish-speaking patients feel heard and supported, providers can guide them toward greater confidence in their treatment decisions, ultimately improving adherence and outcomes.

## 15.3 Using Motivational Interviewing Techniques in Spanish

Motivational interviewing is a patient-centered counseling approach that fosters collaboration, draws out the patient's own motivations for change, and supports autonomy. It is especially powerful when working with Spanish-speaking patients, as it allows them to express their personal values, challenges, and readiness for change in their own words. By respectfully guiding the conversation, healthcare providers can help patients strengthen their confidence and commitment to healthier behaviors.

### 1 Eliciting the Patient's Goals and Motivations

Begin by inviting the patient to identify what changes they might like to make. This empowers the patient and frames the conversation as a partnership rather than a lecture.

For instance, you might say:

- *¿Qué le gustaría cambiar en su salud?* — What would you like to change about your health?
- *¿Tiene alguna motivación para hacer cambios en su estilo de vida, tratamiento o considerar una cirugía?* — Do you have any motivation to make changes in your lifestyle, treatment, or consider surgery?
- *¿Cuáles son sus metas en salud para los próximos 6 meses?* — What are your health goals for the next 6 months?

### 2 Assessing Importance and Readiness for Change

Use scaling questions to help patients evaluate how important change is to them and how confident they feel about making changes. This helps identify barriers and support planning.

Phrases you can use to explain this to the patient:

- *¿Qué tan importante es esto para usted en una escala del uno al diez?* — How important is this to you on a scale of one to ten?

- *¿Qué tan seguro se siente de poder lograrlo?* — How confident do you feel you can achieve it?

- *¿Qué necesitaría para sentirse más seguro de poder lograrlo?* — What would you need to feel more confident about achieving it?

- *¿En qué medida lo que está haciendo actualmente lo está acercando o alejando de lo que quiere lograr en su salud?* — To what extent is what you're currently doing bringing you closer to or further from your health goals?

### 3 Encouraging Problem-Solving and Self-Efficacy

Guide patients in identifying their own solutions and building confidence in their ability to succeed. The goal is to support their autonomy while offering professional guidance.

Example Phrases:

- *¿Qué cree que puede hacer para mejorar su situación?* — What do you think you can do to improve your situation?

- *¿Qué estrategias le han funcionado en el pasado en situaciones parecidas?* — What strategies have worked for you in similar situations before?

- *¿En quién podría apoyarse para llevar a cabo este cambio?* — Who could you rely on to help you make this change?

### 4 Best Practices for Motivational Interviewing

- Avoid arguing or correcting; use reflective listening.
- Reinforce the patient's strengths and previous successes.
- Summarize key points to ensure mutual understanding.
- Respect the patient's pace and readiness to change.
- Offer ongoing support and follow-up opportunities.
- Help the patient explore the discrepancy between their goals and current behavior.

Motivational interviewing in Spanish creates space for patients to share their personal reasons for change and strengthens their confidence in taking action. By using these techniques with empathy and cultural sensitivity, healthcare providers can support long-lasting behavioral change and better health outcomes in Spanish-speaking communities.

## 15.4 Supporting Patient Adherence to Treatment Plans

Supporting patients in following their treatment plans is a key element of successful healthcare outcomes. Spanish-speaking patients may face various cultural, financial, or logistical barriers that interfere with adherence. Effective counseling requires not only providing clear instructions but also collaborating with patients to find obstacles and create practical solutions.

## 1 Exploring Barriers to Adherence

Start by inviting patients to share any concerns or difficulties they may encounter in following their treatment plan. This helps uncover challenges that may not be immediately obvious.

Sample questions for gathering information:

- *¿Qué obstáculos tiene para seguir el tratamiento?* — What challenges do you face in following the treatment?

- *¿Qué retos anticipa y cómo podría superarlos?* — What challenges do you anticipate, and how might you overcome them?

- *¿Hay algo que le impida tomar los medicamentos según lo indicado?* — Is there anything preventing you from taking the medications as prescribed?

## 2 Collaborating on Solutions

Collaborate with the patient to find realistic strategies to overcome obstacles. Shared problem-solving empowers patients and increases commitment to the treatment plan.

Model phrases :

- *Podemos encontrar soluciones juntos.* — We can find solutions together.

- *Hablemos de lo que funcionaría mejor para usted.* — Let's talk about what would work best for you.

- *¿Por cuál de los cambios que hablamos le gustaría empezar?* — Which of the changes we discussed would you like to start with?

## 3 Offering Ongoing Encouragement and Support

Reinforce the importance of adherence while reassuring patients that they have support throughout the process. Positive reinforcement builds confidence and trust.

Model phrases :

- *Queremos acompañarle en este proceso, paso a paso.* — We want to support you through this process, step by step.

- *Lo que decida, seguimos aquí para ayudarle a alcanzar sus objetivos de salud.* — Whatever you decide, we're still here to help you reach your health goals.

## 4 Best Practices for Supporting Adherence

- Provide clear, written instructions in Spanish.
- Use simple language and confirm understanding.
- Involve family members or caregivers when appropriate.
- Schedule regular follow-ups to monitor progress.
- Acknowledge successes and offer ongoing encouragement.

Supporting patient adherence to treatment plans requires both clinical guidance and emotional support. By using patient-centered communication in Spanish, healthcare providers can help patients feel empowered, motivated, and capable of successfully managing their health conditions.

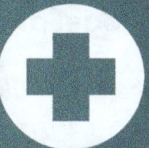

## CHAPTER 16

# EXPLAINING THE HEALTHCARE SYSTEM TO SPANISH-SPEAKING PATIENTS

## 16.1 Explaining Different Types of Healthcare Providers and Settings

Navigating the healthcare system can be confusing for any patient, and even more so for Spanish-speaking patients who may face language, cultural, or systemic barriers. By clearly explaining the several types of healthcare providers and settings, healthcare professionals can help patients understand where to seek care, build trust in the system, and feel more confident managing their health needs.

### 1  Explaining the Role of the Primary Care Provider

Primary care providers are often the patient's main point of contact for routine check-ups, preventive care, and management of chronic conditions. It is important that patients understand the value of having a regular primary care provider.

Model phrases you can use:

- ⊙ *Su médico de atención primaria es quien se encarga de su cuidado general.* — Your primary care doctor is responsible for your overall care.

- ⊙ *Él o ella coordina su cuidado y lo remitirá a otros especialistas si es necesario.* — He or she coordinates your care and refers you to other specialists if needed.

- ⊙ *Su médico de atención primaria es su primer punto de contacto para cualquier inquietud de salud.* — Your primary care doctor is your first point of contact for any health concerns.

### 2  Clarifying Emergency Room Services

Patients should understand that the emergency room is intended for conditions that are life-threatening or require immediate medical attention. Access to care is determined through a triage process, which assesses, characterizes, and categorizes the severity of each patient's condition in order to prioritize care based on urgency.

Model phrases you can use:

- *En el área de Urgencias atendemos situaciones graves que requieren atención médica inmediata.* — In the emergency room, we treat serious conditions that require immediate medical attention.

- *Si presenta un problema grave y repentino, debe acudir a Urgencias.* — If you experience a sudden and serious condition, go to the emergency department right away.

- *En Urgencia se prioriza para los casos que representan un riesgo inmediato para la vida o la salud.* — In the emergency department, care is prioritized for cases that pose an immediate risk to life or health.

- *En la Urgencia, los pacientes no siempre son atendidos en el orden de llegada, sino según la urgencia médica.* — In the Emergency Room, patients are seen based on the severity of their condition, not necessarily the order of arrival.

### 3  Describing the Role of Specialists

- Specialists provide focused care for specific health conditions. Helping patients understand the role of specialists builds confidence in following through with referrals and specialized treatments.

- For instance, some common phrases include:

- *En nuestro hospital contamos con varias especialidades, como cardiología, neurología o endocrinología, entre otras.* — Our hospital offers several specialties, such as cardiology, neurology, or endocrinology, among others.

- *Los especialistas trabajan en conjunto con su médico principal para brindarle una atención integral.* — Specialists work alongside your primary doctor to provide comprehensive care.

- *Su médico de atención primaria puede referirlo a un especialista según sea necesario.* — Your primary care doctor may refer you to a specialist as needed.

### 4  Best Practices for Explaining Healthcare Roles

- Use simple, patient-friendly language in Spanish.
- Provide examples of common situations for each type of care.
- Offer printed guides or charts that map out the healthcare system.
- Reassure patients that they can ask questions anytime.
- Clarify when to seek care from a primary doctor versus going to the emergency room.

## 16.2 Explaining Insurance and Payment Processes

Understanding insurance and payment systems can be one of the most stressful and confusing aspects of healthcare for Spanish-speaking patients. Language barriers, unfamiliar terminology, and financial concerns often create additional anxiety. Healthcare providers and staff can greatly reduce this stress by using simple, patient-friendly language and offering supportive guidance through the financial aspects of care.

### 1 Explaining Insurance Coverage

Begin by clearly explaining what the patient's insurance will cover and what portion, if any, they may be responsible for paying. Reassure patients that help is available to answer questions.

For example, you might say

- *Su seguro cubre parte del costo.* — Your insurance covers part of the cost.
- *Verificaremos su cobertura antes del procedimiento.* — We will verify your coverage before the procedure.
- *Si su plan no cubre el servicio, le informaremos antes de continuar.* — If your plan doesn't cover the service, we will let you know before proceeding.
- *Podemos ayudarle a entender lo que cubre su seguro y responder sus preguntas.* — We can help you understand what your insurance covers and answer any questions you may have.
- *Algunos procedimientos requieren autorización previa por parte de su aseguradora.* — Some procedures require prior authorization from your insurance provider.

### 2 Clarifying Copays, Deductibles, and Out-of-Pocket Costs

Use simple examples to explain common insurance terms like copays and deductibles, which may be unfamiliar to many patients.

Example Phrase:

- *Dependiendo de su plan, es posible que tenga que pagar un copago o un deducible.* — Depending on your plan, you may have to pay a copay or deductible.
- *El copago es una cantidad fija que usted paga por cada visita o servicio.* — The copay is a fixed amount you pay for each visit or service.
- *El deducible es la cantidad que debe pagar antes de que su seguro cubra el resto.* — The deductible is the amount you must pay before your insurance covers the rest.
- *El costo de su bolsillo es el total que debe pagar usted mismo, sin que lo cubra el seguro.* — The out-of-pocket cost is the total amount you must pay yourself, not covered by insurance.

### 3 Offering Billing Assistance and Financial Counseling

Reassure patients that billing staff are available to help explain the charges, review statements, and explore payment options if needed.

One common way to say it is:

- *Podemos ayudarle a entender su factura.* — *We can help you understand your bill.*
- *Si tiene preguntas sobre el costo, por favor hable con nuestro personal de facturación.* — If you have questions about the cost, please speak with our billing staff.

- *Ofrecemos orientación financiera para ayudarle a manejar los costos del tratamiento.* — We offer financial counseling to help you manage the cost of treatment.
- *¿Necesita ayuda para establecer un plan de pago?* — Do you need help setting up a payment plan?

**4 Best Practices for Explaining Insurance and Payments**

- Avoid technical insurance jargon.
- Use visual aids or handouts to explain billing processes.
- Offer written estimates of costs whenever possible.
- Encourage patients to ask questions and verify understanding.
- Be sensitive to financial concerns and explore available assistance programs.

## 16.3 Guiding Patients Through Referrals and Appointments

Navigating referrals and scheduling appointments can be especially challenging for Spanish-speaking patients due to language barriers, unfamiliar healthcare systems, and uncertainty about the process. Healthcare providers play a critical role in offering clear instructions and practical assistance to ensure patients successfully follow through with needed care.

**1 Explaining the Referral Process**

When referring a patient to a specialist or additional services, explain why the referral is necessary and how the process works. This helps build trust and reduces anxiety about seeing a new provider.

In Spanish, you could ask:

- *Le vamos a referir / remitir a un especialista.* — We will arrange a referral to a specialist for you.
- *Lo vamos a trasladar a otra institución de mayor complejidad* — We are going to transfer you to a higher-level care facility.
- *El especialista evaluará su condición más a fondo.* — The specialist will evaluate your condition further.
- *Por su condición clínica, haremos su traslado en una ambulancia.* — Due to your medical condition, we will transfer you by ambulance.

**2 Providing Contact Information and Appointment Details**

Offer patients written instructions with clear information about the location, contact details, and any preparation required for the appointment.

In Spanish, you could ask:

- *Esta es la dirección y el número telefónico de la clínica.* — This is the address and phone number of the clinic.

- *Debe llegar 15 minutos antes de su cita.* — You should arrive 15 minutes before your appointment.

- *Recuerde que nuestro centro de atención lo atiende 24 horas los 7 días de la semana en este número.* — Remember that our support center is available 24/7 at this number.

- *Los siguientes son nuestros puntos de contacto para usted.* — Here are the ways you can reach us.

- *Puede consultar su información médica y programar sus citas a través de nuestra página web o de la app de la clínica.* — You can access your medical information and schedule your appointments through our website or the clinic's app.

## 3  Helping with Scheduling and Coordination

Some patients may need help navigating scheduling systems, especially if they are not fluent in English or familiar with online systems. Offer assistance to make the process as smooth as possible.

One common way to say it is:

- *Si necesita ayuda para programar la cita, avísenos.* — If you need help scheduling the appointment, let us know.

- *Nuestro personal puede hacer la cita por usted si lo desea.* — Our staff can make the appointment for you if you wish.

- *Con gusto te ayudamos a agendar tu cita, solo llámanos.* — We're happy to help you schedule your visit—just give us a call.

## 4  Best Practices for Supporting Referrals and Appointments

- Provide written instructions in Spanish.
- Confirm the patient understands where to go and whom to see.
- Offer interpreter services when needed.
- Follow up after the referral to ensure the appointment was scheduled.
- Remind patients of upcoming appointments through calls or text messages.

Supporting Spanish-speaking patients through referrals and appointments ensures they can access the full spectrum of healthcare services. Clear communication, written instructions, and personalized assistance help patients feel supported and confident as they navigate the healthcare system. It is essential to offer all the available options the institution provides for contacting them, including an orientation or customer service area that can assist with guidance and help resolve any concerns.

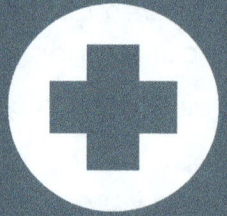

BOOK 7

# THE HEALTHCARE PROFESSIONAL'S
# SPANISH REFERENCE

## A GUIDE TO MEDICAL ABBREVIATIONS, KEY RESOURCES, AND CONTINUED LEARNING FOR PATIENT CARE

ACQUIRE A LOT

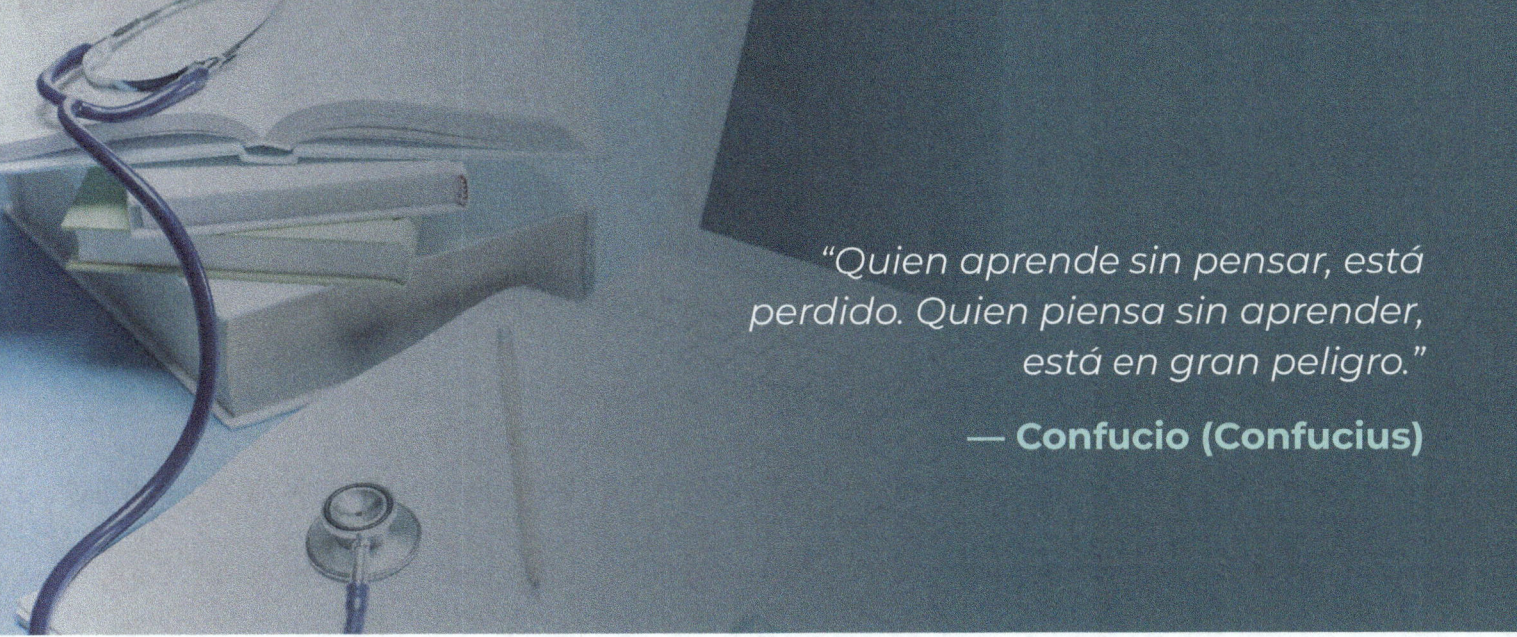

*"Quien aprende sin pensar, está perdido. Quien piensa sin aprender, está en gran peligro."*

**— Confucio (Confucius)**

## CHAPTER 17

# UNDERSTANDING COMMON CULTURAL BELIEFS AND PRACTICES RELATED TO HEALTH

## 17.1 Family-Centered Decision-Making

In many Hispanic and Latino cultures, healthcare decisions are often made collectively with the involvement of family members. Patients may defer to spouses, parents, children, or extended family members when discussing diagnoses and treatment options.

**1  Cultural Insights:**

- Family support can provide emotional strength but may also delay individual decision-making.

- Providers should involve family members as appropriate while ensuring the patient's autonomy is respected.

- Asking permission to include family in discussions demonstrates cultural sensitivity.

- In some cultures, medical decisions are made by the family rather than the individual, and it is often the father who takes the lead in making these decisions. It is important to be aware that these choices may also be influenced by spiritual or religious beliefs, which providers should acknowledge with sensitivity

**2  Traditional Remedies and Folk Healers**

Many Spanish-speaking patients may use home remedies, herbal treatments, or consult traditional healers such as "curanderos" / "brujos" (healers), "sobadores" / "sobanderos" (traditional massage therapists), or "espiritistas" (spiritual healers). These practices may be used alongside, rather than instead of, Western medicine.

Guidance for Cross-Cultural Interaction:

- Patients may hesitate to disclose alternative treatments unless asked in a non-judgmental way.
- Acknowledge these practices respectfully and assess for potential interactions with prescribed treatments.
- Open dialogue allows providers to educate patients on safe use without dismissing cultural beliefs.
- A good practice is to remain open to the possibility that the patient may have first sought care from folk healers or traditional remedies and to explore the implications this may have for their health and treatment.

### 3  Spiritual Beliefs and Interpretations of Illness

Spirituality often plays a significant role in how patients understand illness and healing. Some cultural interpretations may involve beliefs in *susto* (soul loss due to fright), *mal de* ojo (evil eye), or divine will.

It can be very helpful to ask:

- *¿Hay algo importante relacionado con su cultura o creencias que le gustaría que respetáramos durante su atención médica?* — Is there anything important about your culture or beliefs that you would like us to respect during your medical care?

Guidance for Cross-Cultural Interaction:

- In some cultural groups, illness may be viewed as a test, a punishment, or part of God's plan.
- Providers should approach these beliefs with empathy, avoiding contradiction or confrontation.
- Integrating spiritual support, such as pastoral care or prayer, may enhance the patient's comfort and trust.
- It is advisable to ask the patient whether they would like to receive any form of spiritual support during their care.

### 4  Best Practices for Recognizing Cultural Beliefs

- Ask open-ended questions about health beliefs and practices.
- Show curiosity rather than skepticism when learning about cultural traditions.
- Avoid assumptions; every patient is unique even within a shared culture.
- Involve culturally competent interpreters when needed.
- Build long-term trust through respectful, patient-centered dialogue.

By recognizing and respecting the diverse cultural beliefs of Spanish-speaking patients, healthcare providers create a foundation for more effective, Care rooted in respect and kindness. Cultural competence strengthens the therapeutic alliance, reduces misunderstandings, and empowers patients to participate fully in their treatment while honoring their values and traditions.

## 17.2 Recognizing Potential Communication Barriers and How to Overcome Them

For Spanish-speaking patients, these challenges may include language proficiency, differing expectations of care, and health literacy gaps. Recognizing and proactively addressing these barriers enables healthcare providers to deliver safer, more effective, and culturally sensitive care.

### 1 Language Proficiency

Patients with limited English proficiency (LEP) may struggle to fully understand medical discussions, particularly when complex terminology or rapid explanations are used. Professional medical interpreters should always be offered to ensure accurate and complete communication.

Key Considerations:

- Avoid using family members as interpreters, as this can lead to errors or uncomfortable situations.
- Use trained, professional interpreters who understand both language and medical terminology.
- Speak in short, simple sentences and pause frequently to allow interpretation.

How to word it:

- *Si lo necesita, podemos contar con un intérprete profesional para apoyarlo.* — If you need one, we can provide a professional interpreter to assist you.
- *Percibo que la comunicación podría estar siendo un poco difícil. ¿Le ayudaría si traemos a un intérprete profesional?* — I sense that communicating might be a bit challenging, would it help if we brought in a professional interpreter?

### 2 Health Literacy

Some Spanish-speaking patients may have limited familiarity with medical language or the structure of the U.S. healthcare system. Using plain, accessible language and confirming understanding helps ensure patients grasp critical information.

Key Strategies:

- Avoid medical jargon; use simple, everyday words.
- Explain healthcare processes step-by-step.
- Use the "teach-back" method, asking patients to repeat instructions in their own words.
- Provide written materials in plain Spanish with visuals when possible.

How to word it:

- ⊙ *¿Puede explicarme lo que entendió para asegurarme de que lo expliqué claramente? —* Can you explain to me what you understood so I can be sure I explained it clearly?

### 3  Nonverbal Communication

Body language, eye contact, tone of voice, and gestures can all carry different meanings across cultures. Being mindful of nonverbal cues helps avoid misunderstandings and fosters a respectful, comfortable environment.

Key Considerations:

- ⊙ Respect personal space preferences; some patients may feel uncomfortable with proximity.
- ⊙ Avoid gestures or expressions that may have unintended cultural meanings.
- ⊙ Use open, warm facial expressions and calm tone to convey empathy and professionalism.

### 4  Best Practices for Overcoming Communication Barriers

- ⊙ Always assess whether language services are needed.
- ⊙ Simplify complex information and verify understanding.
- ⊙ Remain patient, flexible, and culturally aware.
- ⊙ Encourage questions and reassure patients that it is okay to ask for clarification.
- ⊙ Collaborate with culturally competent staff whenever possible.

Overcoming communication barriers in cross-cultural healthcare requires intentional, respectful, and patient-centered communication strategies. By recognizing the potential for language, literacy, and cultural misunderstandings, healthcare providers can build stronger relationships, improve patient safety, and ensure that every Spanish-speaking patient receives an equitable and caring approach that prioritizes your comfort and autonomy.

## 17.3 Showing Respect for Patient Customs and Traditions

Respecting the cultural customs and traditions of Spanish-speaking patients is essential for building trust, enhancing communication, and delivering high-quality, patient-centered care. Cultural competence goes beyond language proficiency and requires healthcare providers to demonstrate cultural humility, ask thoughtful questions, and adapt care practices to honor the patient's beliefs and values. Even simple gestures of respect can greatly reduce anxiety, foster cooperation, and improve adherence to treatment plans.

### 1  Asking Respectfully About Cultural or Religious Practices

Begin by inviting patients to share any cultural or religious preferences that may affect their care. This demonstrates openness and builds trust from the outset.

Example Phrases and Tips:

- *¿Tiene alguna práctica cultural o religiosa que debamos conocer mientras lo atendemos?* — Do you have any cultural or religious practices we should be aware of while caring for you?

- *¿Hay algo que pueda hacer para que el examen físico sea más cómodo?* — Is there anything I can do to make your physical exam more comfortable?

- *¿Cree que esta recomendación médica podría entrar en conflicto con alguna de sus prácticas religiosas o culturales? Podemos buscar juntos una alternativa.* — Do you think this medical recommendation might conflict with any of your religious or cultural practices? We can work together to find an alternative.

- *¿Ha tenido alguna experiencia negativa con el sistema de salud que le gustaría compartir conmigo o con alguien del equipo de salud?* — Have you had any negative experiences with the healthcare system that you'd like to share with me or with someone from the care team?

### 2  Honoring Modesty and Privacy

For many Spanish-speaking patients, modesty is an important value, especially during physical examinations or personal care. Offering same-gender providers and explaining procedures in advance can reduce discomfort and anxiety.

Key Strategies:

- When possible, offer same-gender providers or chaperones for sensitive exams.
- Explain each step of the examination before proceeding.
- Ensure privacy and allow patients to remain as covered as possible during examinations.

### 3  Acknowledging Dietary and Religious Practices

Many patients may observe dietary restrictions or fasting related to religious beliefs. Providers should inquire respectfully to avoid inadvertently recommending treatments or schedules that conflict with these practices.

Key Strategies:

- Ask if patients observe any fasting periods or dietary restrictions.
- Accommodate sacred days or religious holidays when scheduling appointments, procedures, or hospitalizations.
- Collaborate with nutrition services to offer culturally appropriate meal options.

### 4  Best Practices for Respecting Customs and Traditions

- Approach all discussions with humility and curiosity.
- Avoid making assumptions based on appearance or background.
- Incorporate cultural questions as a routine part of medical history.

- ⊙ Document patient preferences in the medical record.
- ⊙ Encourage ongoing staff training on cultural humility and inclusive communication.

Cultural sensitivity is built on a foundation of respect, open communication, and willingness to adapt care to meet the needs of each patient. By recognizing and honoring the customs and traditions of Spanish-speaking patients, healthcare providers strengthen therapeutic relationships, reduce resistance to care, and create a healthcare environment where all patients feel valued, safe, and respected.

## 17.4 Avoiding Stereotypes and Making Culturally Sensitive Inquiries

Cultural competence involves both understanding general cultural tendencies and recognizing that every patient is an individual with unique experiences, beliefs, and values. While cultural awareness provides helpful context, healthcare providers need to avoid stereotyping or making assumptions based solely on a patient's ethnicity, language, or appearance. By using culturally sensitive inquiry, providers can foster open, respectful dialogue that honors each patient's personal perspective.

### 1 Avoid Assumptions About Patients

Stereotypes can inadvertently lead to misunderstandings or diminished trust. Avoid assuming that a patient's cultural background automatically dictates their beliefs, language skills, or healthcare preferences.

Key Strategies:

- ⊙ Do not presume language fluency, family structure, or religious views.
- ⊙ Allow the patient to share their own background and preferences.
- ⊙ Adapt care based on the patient's specific needs, not perceived norms.

### 2 Use Open-Ended, Culturally Sensitive Questions

Open-ended questions invite patients to share information about their beliefs, concerns, and expectations without leading or judging. This allows providers to gather valuable insight while respecting the patient's autonomy.

Useful expressions when collecting patient information:

- ⊙ *¿Puede contarme cómo ve esta enfermedad?* — Can you tell me more about how you view this illness?
- ⊙ *¿Qué inquietudes tiene sobre el plan de tratamiento?* — What concerns do you have about the treatment plan?
- ⊙ *¿Hay algo culturalmente importante que debamos considerar?* — Is there anything culturally important we should consider?

### 3  Demonstrate Cultural Humility

Cultural humility involves acknowledging that providers are not experts on every patient's culture. Demonstrating curiosity and willingness to learn fosters respect and partnership.

Key Strategies:

- Acknowledge limitations: "I may not be familiar with all aspects of your culture, but I'm eager to learn."
- Listen actively and nonjudgmentally.
- Allow patients to educate providers about their cultural preferences when appropriate.

### 4  Best Practices for Avoiding Stereotypes

- Treat each patient as an individual first.
- Use cultural knowledge as a guide, not a rule.
- Ask questions with genuine curiosity and empathy.
- Document specific patient preferences for future care.
- Provide ongoing staff training in cultural humility.

Avoiding stereotypes and making culturally sensitive inquiries are central to building trust and delivering personalized care. By combining cultural knowledge with respectful, patient-centered dialogue, healthcare providers can ensure that Spanish-speaking patients feel seen, heard, and valued as individuals throughout the healthcare journey.

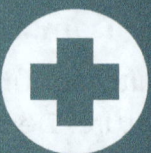

## CHAPTER 18

# COMMON MEDICAL ABBREVIATIONS AND ACRONYMS IN SPANISH

In clinical practice, healthcare professionals frequently rely on abbreviations and acronyms to document patient care quickly and efficiently. For those working with Spanish-speaking patients, understanding common medical abbreviations in Spanish is essential for accurate charting, interpretation of medical records, and effective communication among healthcare team members. This knowledge ensures clarity in documentation and helps avoid errors that may arise from language differences or translation inconsistencies.

### Common Medical Abbreviations

| Abreviatura / Abbreviation | Español / Spanish | English / Inglés |
|---|---|---|
| AVC | Accidente Vascular Cerebral (sinónimo de ACV) | Cerebrovascular Accident (CVA) |
| AVP | Accidente Vascular Periférico | Peripheral Vascular Accident |
| BK | Bacilo de Koch | Koch's Bacillus / Mycobacterium tuberculosis |
| BUN | Nitrógeno Ureico | Blood Urea Nitrogen (BUN) |
| Bx | Biopsia | Biopsy |
| BZD | Benzodiazepinas | Benzodiazepines |
| CAE | Conducto Auditivo Externo | External Auditory Canal |
| CC or C/C | Cuadro Clínico | Clinical Picture / Clinical Presentation |
| CI | Contraindicación | Contraindication |

| Abreviatura / Abbreviation | Español / Spanish | English / Inglés |
|---|---|---|
| CM | Centímetros | Centimeters |
| Cx or Qx | Cirugía | Surgery |
| DM | Diabetes Mellitus | Diabetes Mellitus |
| Dx | Diagnóstico | Diagnosis |
| ECG or EKG | Electrocardiograma | Electrocardiogram (ECG or EKG) |
| EEG | Electroencefalograma | Electroencephalogram |
| EPOC | Enfermedad Pulmonar Obstructiva Crónica | Chronic Obstructive Pulmonary Disease (COPD) |
| EV or IV | Endovenosa / Intravenosa | Intravenous (IV) |
| FA | Fibrilación Auricular (dependiendo del contexto) | Atrial Fibrillation (context-dependent) |
| FA | Fosfatasa Alcalina (dependiendo del contexto) | Alkaline Phosphatase (context-dependent) |
| FC | Frecuencia Cardíaca | Heart Rate (HR) |
| FEVI | Fracción de Eyección del Ventrículo Izquierdo | Left Ventricular Ejection Fraction (LVEF) |
| FR | Frecuencia Respiratoria | Respiratory Rate (RR) |
| FUR or FUM | Fecha de última regla / menstruación | Last Menstrual Period (LMP) |
| GB | Glóbulos Blancos | White Blood Cells (WBCs) |
| GPC | Guía de Práctica Clínica | Clinical Practice Guideline (CPG) |
| GRE | Glóbulos Rojos Empacados | Packed Red Blood Cells (PRBCs) |
| HB | Hemoglobina | Hemoglobin (Hb) |
| HC | Historia Clínica | Medical History / Clinical Record |
| HCTO | Hematocrito | Hematocrit (Hct) |
| HIC | Hipertensión Intracraneal | Intracranial Hypertension |
| HTA | Hipertensión Arterial | High Blood Pressure |

| Abreviatura / Abbreviation | Español / Spanish | English / Inglés |
| --- | --- | --- |
| HTP | Hipertensión Pulmonar / Portal | Pulmonary / Portal Hypertension (context-dependent) |
| IAM | Infarto Agudo de Miocardio | Acute Myocardial Infarction (AMI) |
| IMC | Índice de Masa Corporal | Body Mass Index (BMI) |
| IOT | Intubación Orotraqueal | Orotracheal Intubation |
| ITU or IVU | Infección del tracto urinario / vías urinarias | Urinary Tract Infection (UTI) |
| LCR | Líquido Cefalorraquídeo | Cerebrospinal Fluid (CSF) |
| LES | Lupus Eritematoso Sistémico | Systemic Lupus Erythematosus (SLE) |
| NA | No Aplica | Not Applicable (N/A) |
| NPT | Nutrición Parenteral Total | Total Parenteral Nutrition (TPN) |
| OD | Ojo Derecho / Oído Derecho | Right Eye / Right Ear (context-dependent) |
| OI | Ojo Izquierdo / Oído Izquierdo | Left Eye / Left Ear (context-dependent) |
| PCR | Proteína C Reactiva | C-Reactive Protein (CRP) |
| Px | Pronóstico | Prognosis |
| RM | Resonancia Magnética | Magnetic Resonance Imaging (MRI) |
| Rx | Radiografía / Receta | X-ray / Prescription (context-dependent) |
| SAO2 | Saturación Arterial de Oxígeno | Arterial Oxygen Saturation (SaO$_2$) |
| SC | Subcutáneo | Subcutaneous (SC) |
| SCA | Síndrome Coronario Agudo | Acute Coronary Syndrome (ACS) |
| SS | Se Solicita | Requested |
| T or (T°) | Temperatura Corporal | Body Temperature (T°) |
| TA | Tensión Arterial | Blood Pressure (BP) |

| Abreviatura / Abbreviation | Español / Spanish | English / Inglés |
|---|---|---|
| TAM | Tensión Arterial Media | Mean Arterial Pressure |
| TBC | Tuberculosis | Tuberculosis (TB) |
| TP | Tiempo de Protrombina | Prothrombin Time |
| TPT | Tiempo de Tromboplastina Parcial Activada | Activated Partial Thromboplastin Time |
| VO | Vía Oral | Oral Route |
| VSG | Velocidad de Sedimentación Globular | Erythrocyte Sedimentation Rate (ESR) |

## 1 Best Practices for Using Medical Abbreviations

- ⊙ Always ensure all healthcare team members are familiar with the abbreviations in use.
- ⊙ Avoid introducing non-standard abbreviations to prevent confusion, in line with the Joint Commission's recommendations for improving patient safety and communication
- ⊙ When communicating with patients, avoid abbreviations and explain terms in full.
- ⊙ Provide training and reference materials for staff who work with Spanish-language medical documentation.

Mastering common medical abbreviations in Spanish enhances efficiency, reduces misunderstandings, and ensures continuity of care for Spanish-speaking patients. Healthcare providers who are fluent in both the language and documentation practices of Spanish-speaking populations are better equipped to deliver safe, effective, and culturally competent care.

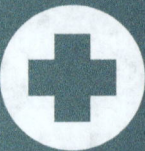

CHAPTER 19

# TRUSTED SPANISH-LANGUAGE RESOURCES FOR HEALTHCARE PROFESSIONALS

Access to reliable, high-quality Spanish-language resources is essential for healthcare professionals who care for Spanish-speaking patients. These resources help clinicians strengthen their medical Spanish skills, stay informed about public health updates, and provide culturally appropriate patient education. The following curated list includes trusted organizations, websites, and educational platforms that support both professional development and patient-centered care.

### 1  Bilingual Patient Education Resources

These platforms provide comprehensive, easy-to-understand materials for patient education:

- "MedlinePlus en español": (https://medlineplus.gov/spanish/): It is a health information service for patients, families, and friends. It is produced by the U.S. National Library of Medicine (NLM).

- "CDC en español" (https://www.cdc.gov/spanish): Public health guidance, vaccine updates, infectious disease information, and prevention guidelines in Spanish.

- Scielo ( https://scielo.isciii.es/scielo.php): Virtual library consisting of a collection of Spanish scientific journals in the health sciences. It is the result of a collaboration between BIREME (Latin American and Caribbean Center on Health Sciences Information), FAPESP (São Paulo Research Foundation) and Spain's National Library of Health Sciences.

- MEDES – "MEDicina en Español" (https://www.fundacionlilly.com/impulso-medicina/medes): Page of the Lilly Foundation to promote the use of Spanish as a language for the transmission of scientific knowledge in general, and of health sciences in particular.

- WebMD: (https://www.webmd.com: Through its section WEBMD *en Español*, it provides reliable medical and health information about diseases, treatments and symptoms, healthy living, medications, and wellness.

## 2 · Programs Supporting Spanish-speaking Patients

These organizations help facilitate healthcare access and culturally sensitive services for Spanish-speaking communities:

- Medi-Cal Access Program (MCAP): Health services for Spanish-speaking patients in California, including prenatal care and insurance support.
- National Hispanic Medical Association (NHMA): Professional organization offering resources for Latino healthcare providers, cultural competency training, and policy advocacy.
- National Alliance for Hispanic Health and the Hispanic Federation are both prominent organizations dedicated to improving the well-being of Hispanic communities in the United States.
- Migrant Clinicians Network (Health Network): Provides case navigation, medical record transfers, and continuity of care for mobile Latino patients, particularly those with chronic illnesses and who cross borders.
- Health Initiative of the Americas (HIA) – UC Berkeley: An academic program that leads research, education, and outreach aimed at improving the health of Latino immigrants in the U.S. and Latin America.
- New York-Presbyterian Hospital: Cultural navigators in emergency services for patients with language barriers, improving appointment scheduling and referrals.

## 3 · Medical Spanish Education for Providers

Healthcare professionals can enhance their ability to communicate effectively with Spanish-speaking patients by enrolling in specialized medical Spanish programs. Below are some reputable options available:

- Canopy Learn: Medical Spanish training modules designed for healthcare professionals to improve communication with Spanish-speaking patients.
- Spanish for Healthcare Professionals – UC San Diego.
- Medical Spanish Courses – Boston Medical Spanish Center.
- New York Institute of Technology – Spanish for Healthcare Workers.
- City University of New York – Spanish for Health Professions.
- University of Miami – Intensive Medical Spanish Program.

## 4 · Best Practices for Using Spanish-Language Resources

- Regularly review and incorporate updated Spanish-language materials into patient care.
- Share patient education materials in both print and digital formats.
- Use professional translation and interpreter services for complex communication.
- Engage in ongoing medical Spanish education to strengthen clinical language skills.

- Verify information through trusted sources to ensure medical accuracy and cultural relevance.

By utilizing high-quality Spanish-language resources, healthcare professionals can better serve Spanish-speaking patients with confidence and cultural sensitivity. These tools not only improve communication but also promote health literacy, trust, and more equitable healthcare outcomes for diverse patient populations.

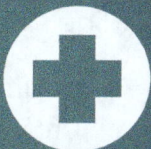

CHAPTER 20

# TIPS FOR CONTINUED LEARNING AND LANGUAGE DEVELOPMENT

Achieving and maintaining proficiency in Medical Spanish is a continuous journey that requires consistent practice, exposure, and a commitment to lifelong learning. For healthcare professionals, strong language skills not only improve patient care but also foster deeper trust and stronger therapeutic relationships with Spanish-speaking patients. This chapter outlines practical strategies and tools for ongoing language development that can fit into any busy healthcare professional's schedule.

**1  Commit to Daily Practice**

Daily, consistent exposure to Spanish is one of the most powerful ways to build lasting language skills. Even short sessions of 15 to 30 minutes can significantly reinforce your vocabulary, grammar, and pronunciation—often more effectively than occasional long study periods. Make Spanish a part of your everyday routine by setting aside a focused time to read a short article, listen to a podcast, or practice speaking aloud. With steady daily practice, you'll build confidence and fluency step by step.

**2  Utilize Mobile Apps and Online Platforms**

Language learning apps and online platforms provide structured lessons, interactive exercises, pronunciation guides, and contextual vocabulary practice. Many also include cultural insights and real-life dialogues, making them ideal for busy professionals, as they can be accessed anytime and adapted to individual learning paces.

Recommended Apps:

- ⊙ Duolingo
- ⊙ Canopy (Medical Spanish Focused)
- ⊙ LingQ

Online Resources:

- ⊙ Coursera (https://www.coursera.org): It includes courses such as "Spanish for Healthcare Professionals" from universities like the University of California and the University of Arizona.
- ⊙ edX (www.edx.org): Courses offered by institutions such as Georgetown University and the Polytechnic University of Valencia (UPV), featuring university-accredited certification.

### 3 Engage in Peer Practice and Language Exchange

Conversing with fluent speakers is one of the most effective ways to build confidence and refine your language skills. Look for opportunities to practice with colleagues, patients (when appropriate), or language partners.

Consider using the following strategies to enhance your conversational skills:

- ⊙ Partner with Spanish-speaking colleagues.
- ⊙ Join language exchange groups or online conversation forums.

### 4 Immerse Yourself Through Spanish Media

Media immersion helps you become familiar with natural language use, regional accents, and practical medical vocabulary in context.

You may want to consider the following:

- ⊙ Watch medical dramas, documentaries, or news programs in Spanish to reinforce real-life vocabulary. Popular medical series like Dr. House, The Resident, Grey's Anatomy, or Boston Med (in Spanish or with Spanish subtitles) can be especially helpful.
- ⊙ Listen to medical podcasts in Spanish during your commute or free time. Some of the more popular are:
  - ◆ Medical Spanish Podcast (by Dr. Molly Martin): Interactive lessons with audio and transcripts.
  - ◆ Learn Medical Spanish: AFP Medical Journal Podcast features summaries of articles from American Family Physician, providing relevant and up-to-date clinical content for healthcare professionals.
  - ◆ "Pediatras en Línea" from the Children's Hospital Colorado: Educational podcast for Spanish-speaking pediatricians.
- ⊙ Instagram Accounts for Medical Spanish:
  - ◆ Medical Spanish Education (@spanishmed_): A platform created by a certified Latina nurse, focused on teaching medical Spanish through visual resources and infographics.
  - ◆ IV Spanish (@ivspanish): Specializes in "Hospital Spanish," teaching useful clinical phrases and vocabulary for professionals, especially with ANKI-style flashcards.

- NAMSpanish (@namspanish): An interdisciplinary group working to improve language proficiency and health equity, with posts focused on health and language.

- Facebook Resources for Medical Spanish

    - Learning Medical Spanish – Group dedicated to professionals sharing resources and engaging in discussion.

    - National Association of Medical Spanish (NAMS) – Professional group for discussion and networking.

- Learn Medical Spanish with Rios Associates – Group focused on training and interactive materials.

## 5  Best Practices for Sustained Progress

- Set measurable short- and long-term learning goals.
- Track vocabulary growth and areas for improvement.
- Schedule periodic assessments to measure progress.
- Incorporate medical Spanish practice into daily patient interactions.
- Celebrate milestones to maintain motivation and engagement.

Mastery of Medical Spanish takes time, consistency, and active engagement. By integrating these strategies into daily routines, healthcare professionals can continuously build confidence, improve fluency, and deliver exceptional, culturally responsive care to Spanish-speaking patients.

Consistent use of these tools ensures better care, reduces disparities, and fosters cultural competence

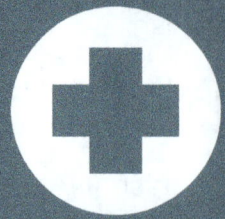

BOOK 8

# SHORT STORIES IN SPANISH FOR HEALTHCARE PROFESSIONALS

## 15 ENGAGING REAL-LIFE STORIES TO BOOST CONFIDENCE AND IMPROVE OUTCOMES WITH SPANISH-SPEAKING PATIENTS

ACQUIRE A LOT

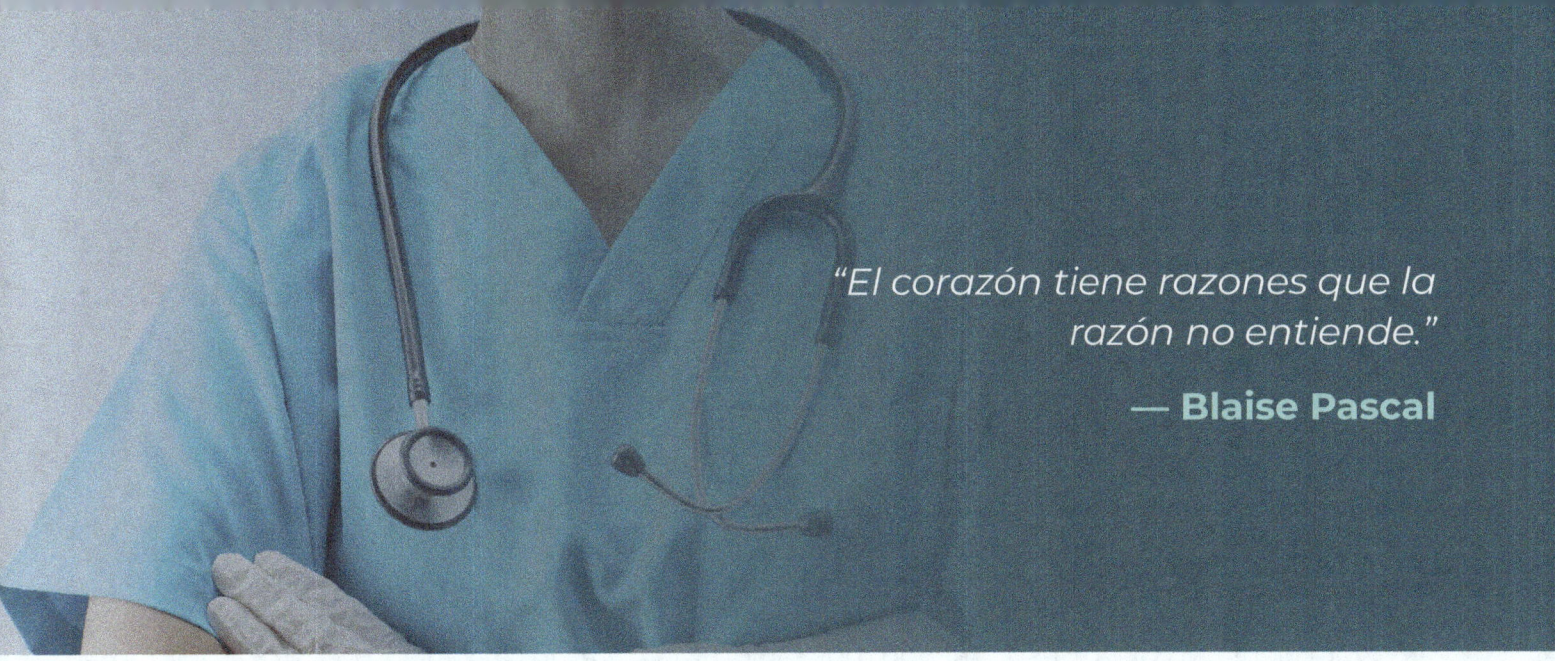

*"El corazón tiene razones que la razón no entiende."*

**— Blaise Pascal**

HISTORIA 1:

# "NO ES 'NERVIOS', ES EL CORAZÓN"

## Un caso de taquicardia en la sala de urgencias

La sala de urgencias del St. Mark's Hospital era un caos controlado, una sinfonía de pitidos de monitores, conversaciones apresuradas y el murmullo constante de la ansiedad. El Dr. Evans, un médico de urgencias con cinco años de experiencia, se sentía cómodo en este entorno, pero aún estaba perfeccionando su español médico, una habilidad cada vez más necesaria en su diversa comunidad.

Su próxima paciente era Elena, una mujer de 52 años sentada en una camilla, con la mirada fija en sus manos. A su lado, su hijo, un joven de unos veinte años llamado Miguel, traducía con nerviosismo.

—She says she's just very nervous, doctor. She thinks it's her nerves —dijo Miguel.

El Dr. Evans asintió, pero observó a Elena. Su piel tenía una ligera palidez y su respiración era un poco más rápida de lo normal. Se dirigió a ella directamente con una voz tranquila.

—Buenas noches, señora Elena. Soy el Dr. Evans. ¿Cómo se siente hoy? —preguntó, usando un tono formal y respetuoso como había aprendido.

Elena levantó la vista, sorprendida de que le hablara en español. —Un poco mareada, doctor. Y siento... como un aleteo aquí —dijo, señalando su pecho.

—Okay, ¿dónde le duele? ¿O es más una molestia?

—No es un dolor, es... raro. Como si mi corazón corriera una carrera. Son los nervios, siempre me pasa cuando me preocupo.

*Short Stories in Spanish for Healthcare Professionals*

183

Miguel intervino de nuevo. —She says it's not pain, just her heart racing. It happens when she worries.

El Dr. Evans sabía que "nervios" era un término muy común en la comunidad hispana para describir una amplia gama de síntomas, desde la ansiedad genuina hasta problemas físicos graves. Ignorarlo sería un error.

—Entiendo. Pero vamos a asegurarnos de que todo esté bien. Le voy a tomar la presión arterial y a revisar sus signos vitales.

La enfermera ya había colocado el manguito. La presión arterial estaba elevada: 150/95 mmHg. La frecuencia cardíaca en el monitor marcaba 160 latidos por minuto, muy por encima de lo normal.

—Señora Elena, su corazón está latiendo muy rápido. Necesitamos hacerle un electrocardiograma, o ECG. Es una prueba rápida que nos muestra la actividad eléctrica de su corazón. No duele nada.

Mientras la enfermera conectaba los electrodos en el pecho, brazos y piernas de Elena, el Dr. Evans continuó hablando con calma para tranquilizarla.

—Solo necesito que se relaje y no se mueva. Respire profundo.

El trazado del ECG apareció en la pantalla. Mostraba una taquicardia supraventricular (TSV), un tipo de arritmia que, aunque no siempre es mortal, necesita tratamiento inmediato para evitar complicaciones. Definitivamente, no eran solo "nervios".

El Dr. Evans se sentó junto a Elena, con el papel del ECG en la mano.

—Bueno, Elena, tenemos el resultado. La prueba muestra que usted tiene una condición llamada taquicardia. Esto significa que la parte superior de su corazón está enviando señales eléctricas demasiado rápido. No es por nerviosismo, es un problema eléctrico que podemos tratar aquí mismo.

Miguel tradujo para asegurarse de que su madre entendiera completamente. La expresión de Elena cambió del nerviosismo a la preocupación.

—¿Y es grave, doctor?

—En este momento, la estamos controlando. Vamos a darle un medicamento por la vía intravenosa para que su corazón vuelva a su ritmo normal. Sentirá algo extraño en el pecho por unos segundos, pero es normal y pasará rápido. No se preocupe, estamos aquí con usted.

Le administraron la adenosina. Tal como el Dr. Evans le advirtió, Elena sintió una breve sensación de opresión en el pecho y el ritmo en el monitor se detuvo por un instante antes de reanudarse a unos saludables 80 latidos por minuto.

Los ojos de Elena se llenaron de lágrimas de alivio. —Ya... ya me siento mejor. Gracias, doctor.

El Dr. Evans sonrió. —Me alegro mucho. Este caso nos enseña algo muy importante. A veces, los "nervios" pueden ser algo más. Usted hizo bien en venir a la sala de emergencias.

## Análisis de la Situación y Puntos Clave

**Nota Cultural y Lingüística:** El término **"nervios"** es un modismo cultural en muchas comunidades hispanas. Puede referirse a estrés, ansiedad, ataques de pánico o, como en este caso, a síntomas físicos como palpitaciones o mareos. Un profesional de la salud no debe descartar los síntomas físicos solo porque el paciente los atribuye a los "nervios". Es crucial investigar la causa subyacente.

### Vocabulario Médico Utilizado:

- **Dolor (Pain)**: El síntoma principal que se debe evaluar.
- **Nervios (Nerves)**: El término cultural clave que puede enmascarar una condición médica.
- **Signos vitales (Vital signs)**: Medidas básicas como la presión arterial y la frecuencia cardíaca.
- **Frecuencia cardíaca (Heart rate)**: El número de veces que el corazón late por minuto.
- **Electrocardiograma (ECG/EKG)**: Una prueba fundamental en cardiología.
- **Vía intravenosa (Intravenous - IV)**: Ruta de administración de medicamentos directamente en una vena.

### Estrategia de Comunicación:

1. **Establecer Confianza:** El Dr. Evans se dirigió a la paciente en su idioma, usando un tono formal y respetuoso (usted), lo que inmediatamente generó una conexión.
2. **No Descartar, Investigar:** En lugar de aceptar la autoevaluación del paciente ("son los nervios"), utilizó esa información como punto de partida para una investigación clínica exhaustiva.
3. **Explicar Procedimientos:** Explicó de manera sencilla qué era un ECG y por qué era necesario, reduciendo el miedo del paciente a lo desconocido.
4. **Comunicar el Diagnóstico con Claridad:** Tradujo un término médico complejo (taquicardia supraventricular) a una explicación simple ("un problema eléctrico") que la paciente pudo entender.
5. Manejar las Expectativas del Tratamiento: Advirtió a la paciente sobre la extraña sensación que provocaría el medicamento, preparándola y evitando que entrara en pánico durante el tratamiento. Esto demuestra un cuidado centrado en el paciente.

# LA RECETA DE LA ABUELA

## Cuando el remedio casero interfiere con la medicación

La clínica comunitaria de Oakwood bullía de actividad. Sarah, una enfermera practicante (NP) dedicada, revisaba la **historia clínica** de su siguiente paciente, el señor Roberto Morales, un hombre de 68 años con **hipertensión** crónica. Sus notas indicaban que, a pesar de haberle recetado lisinopril hacía tres meses, su **presión arterial** seguía peligrosamente alta en su último **chequeo**.

El señor Morales entró al consultorio con una sonrisa amable, pero Sarah notó una pizca de preocupación en sus ojos.

—Buenas tardes, señor Morales. Soy Sarah. ¿Cómo ha estado? —dijo ella en un español claro y pausado.

—Ahí vamos, enfermera. Un poco cansado, pero bien, gracias a Dios.

—Veo en sus registros que su presión sigue un poco alta. **¿Está tomando su medicamento para la presión todos los días?**

—Sí, claro. Todos los días, como usted me dijo. Una pastillita en la mañana.

Sarah sabía que la falta de adherencia era común, pero la respuesta del señor Morales sonaba sincera. Decidió indagar un poco más, recordando que la salud es un concepto integral que a menudo incluye prácticas fuera de la medicina convencional.

—Entiendo. Aparte de la pastilla, **¿está tomando alguna otra cosa?** A veces, las personas toman tés, hierbas o remedios caseros que les han recomendado.

El señor Morales dudó un momento antes de responder. —Bueno... mi esposa me prepara un té que le dio su mamá. Es de "cola de caballo". Dicen que es muy bueno para limpiar los riñones y bajar la presión. Me lo tomo dos veces al día.

Sarah asintió, sin mostrar juicio. Este era el dato que necesitaba. La "cola de caballo" (horsetail) es un diurético natural potente. El lisinopril, el medicamento que le recetó, también tiene efectos sobre los riñones y el balance de fluidos. La combinación podría estar causando un desequilibrio.

—Gracias por decírmelo, señor Morales. Es muy importante que yo sepa todo lo que toma. Las hierbas son medicina también y a veces pueden interferir con las pastillas que recetamos.

Sacó una hoja de papel y dibujó un esquema simple.

—Mire, esta es su pastilla, el lisinopril. Ayuda a que sus **vasos sanguíneos** se relajen para que la presión baje —explicó, dibujando un tubo ancho—. El té de cola de caballo, por otro lado, hace que sus **riñones** eliminen más agua y sal —añadió, dibujando unas gotas saliendo de un frijol que representaba el riñón—. Si toma ambos, sus riñones trabajan demasiado y el cuerpo puede perder demasiado potasio, lo que es peligroso y puede hacer que la presión no se controle bien.

El señor Morales observó el dibujo con gran interés. Era la primera vez que alguien le explicaba las cosas de esa manera.

—Ah, no sabía eso. En mi pueblo, todo el mundo toma hierbas. La receta de la abuela nunca falla.

—Lo entiendo perfectamente —respondió Sarah con empatía—. Y muchas hierbas son maravillosas. Pero cuando se mezclan con **medicamentos** recetados, debemos tener cuidado. No quiero que deje de hacer algo que es importante para su cultura, pero su salud es la prioridad. ¿Qué le parece si hacemos un trato?

Hizo una pausa, asegurándose de tener toda su atención.

—Por las próximas dos semanas, vamos a suspender el té. Solo tome la pastilla que yo le receté. Venga a la clínica en una semana para que le tomemos la presión y otra vez en dos semanas para un **chequeo de seguimiento**. Así podemos ver si es el té lo que está afectando el tratamiento.

El señor Morales lo pensó y luego asintió. —Está bien, enfermera. Haremos la prueba.

Dos semanas después, el señor Morales regresó a la clínica. Su presión arterial había bajado a 130/80 mmHg, un nivel mucho más saludable.

—¡Mire eso! —dijo Sarah, mostrándole el número en el monitor—. Su presión está mucho mejor. Parece que la combinación no era la ideal para usted.

El señor Morales sonrió, esta vez con genuino alivio. —Tenía razón, enfermera. Gracias por explicármelo. A veces, uno no sabe.

## Análisis de la Situación y Puntos Clave

**Nota Cultural y Lingüística:** El uso de **remedios caseros** y **hierbas medicinales** está profundamente arraigado en muchas culturas hispanas. Los pacientes pueden no considerarlos "medicamentos" y, por lo tanto, no mencionarlos a menos que se les pregunte directamente. Es crucial preguntar de manera abierta y sin prejuicios para obtener una **historia clínica** completa. Frases como *"¿Toma algún té, hierba o remedio que le hayan recomendado?"* son más efectivas que un simple *"¿Toma otros medicamentos?"*.

## Vocabulario Médico Utilizado:

- **Hipertensión / Presión arterial (Hypertension / Blood pressure)**: Términos fundamentales en atención primaria.

- **Chequeo / Chequeo de seguimiento (Check-up / Follow-up check-up)**: Citas para monitorear la condición del paciente.

- **Medicamento / Pastilla (Medication / Pill)**: Palabras de uso común.

- **Riñones (Kidneys) / Vasos sanguíneos (Blood vessels)**: Vocabulario anatómico básico para explicar el mecanismo de acción de los fármacos.

- **Historia clínica (Medical history)**: El registro de la salud del paciente.

## Estrategia de Comunicación:

1. **Preguntas Abiertas y sin Juicio:** Sarah no desestimó las creencias del paciente. Su pregunta abierta sobre "tés o hierbas" creó un espacio seguro para que el señor Morales compartiera información que de otro modo habría omitido.

2. **Uso de Ayudas Visuales:** El simple dibujo ayudó a desmitificar la interacción farmacológica, convirtiendo un concepto médico complejo en algo visual y fácil de entender. Esto es especialmente útil para pacientes con diferentes niveles de alfabetización en salud.

3. **Crear una Alianza (Hacer un Trato):** En lugar de ordenar al paciente que dejara el té, Sarah le propuso un "trato" o un experimento. Este enfoque colaborativo respeta la autonomía del paciente y lo convierte en un participante activo de su propio cuidado, lo que aumenta la probabilidad de **adherencia**.

4. **Validación Cultural:** Sarah reconoció la importancia de las tradiciones del paciente ("muchas hierbas son maravillosas") antes de explicar el problema clínico. Esta validación es clave para mantener la confianza.

5. **Seguimiento Cercano:** Programar citas de seguimiento a corto plazo demostró un compromiso con el bienestar del paciente y permitió validar los resultados del cambio en el tratamiento.

# "SOLO UN SUSTO"

## Comprendiendo el trauma cultural en un paciente pediátrico

La Dra. Miller era una pediatra que amaba los rompecabezas. Y cada niño, para ella, era un pequeño y fascinante rompecabezas. Pero Leo, de 4 años, era uno particularmente complejo. Estaba sentado en la camilla, acurrucado en el regazo de su madre, Mariana, con una mirada apática que no correspondía a su edad.

—Cuénteme, Mariana, ¿qué le trae por aquí? —preguntó la Dra. Miller con una sonrisa cálida.

—Es que Leo se cayó en el parque hace dos días, del tobogán —comenzó Mariana, con la voz cargada de angustia—. No se golpeó la cabeza fuerte, no hubo sangre, nada. Pero desde entonces, no es el mismo. No quiere comer, se despierta llorando por la noche y está... como ausente.

A su lado, la abuela del niño, Isabel, asintió con solemnidad y añadió en voz baja, pero firme: —Tiene **susto**, doctora. La caída le robó el alma del cuerpo.

La Dra. Miller había escuchado sobre el **susto** durante su formación. Sabía que era una "enfermedad popular" o un síndrome cultural en muchas comunidades latinoamericanas, una condición en la que se cree que un evento traumático hace que el alma abandone el cuerpo, provocando síntomas físicos y emocionales. Descartarlo sería como descartar la preocupación de la familia.

—Gracias por compartir eso conmigo, Isabel. Es muy importante entender todo lo que está pasando —dijo, validando la perspectiva de la abuela antes de volverse hacia Leo—. Hola, campeón. Soy la Dra. Miller. **Voy a revisarte** para asegurarme de que todo esté bien por dentro, ¿de acuerdo?

Realizó un **examen físico** completo. Revisó sus **pupilas** con una pequeña luz para asegurarse de que reaccionaran correctamente, palpó su **abdomen** y su cabeza buscando signos de **dolor** o **hinchazón**, y evaluó sus **reflejos**. Físicamente, todo parecía normal. No había signos evidentes de una **concusión cerebral** o una lesión interna.

—Bueno, físicamente, Leo parece estar muy bien. No veo ninguna señal de una lesión grave por la caída —explicó a la familia.

La abuela frunció el ceño. —Pero no está bien, doctora. Su espíritu no está aquí. Necesita una **limpia** de una curandera para que su alma regrese.

Aquí estaba el punto crucial. La Dra. Miller sabía que no podía recetar una "limpia", pero tampoco podía ignorar la profunda angustia de la familia, que atribuía los síntomas a una causa espiritual.

—Entiendo su preocupación por su bienestar espiritual —dijo con empatía—. El cuerpo y el espíritu están conectados. Lo que ustedes llaman **susto**, en la medicina a veces lo llamamos un "shock" o trauma emocional después de un evento aterrador. El cuerpo también necesita recuperarse de ese miedo.

Utilizó esta "traducción" cultural para tender un puente entre sus dos mundos.

—Mientras ustedes le ayudan a su espíritu a sentirse seguro de nuevo, yo quiero ayudar a su cuerpo. Vamos a hacer dos cosas. Primero, quiero que vigilen a Leo en casa. Si empieza con **vómitos**, un **dolor de cabeza** muy fuerte, o si lo ven más somnoliento de lo normal o confundido, deben traerlo a la **sala de emergencias** de inmediato. Esas serían señales de que la caída fue más seria de lo que parece.

Le entregó a Mariana una hoja con las instrucciones sobre los signos de alarma de una concusión, escrita en español.

—Segundo —continuó—, para ayudar a su cuerpo a recuperarse del "shock", asegúrense de que descanse mucho. Ofrézcanle sus comidas favoritas, aunque solo coma un poquito. Y lo más importante: muchos abrazos. Necesita sentirse seguro.

La abuela la miró, sus facciones se suavizaron. La doctora no se había burlado de ella. Había escuchado y ofrecido un plan que tenía sentido tanto para el cuerpo como para el alma.

—Haremos eso, doctora —dijo Mariana, sintiéndose visiblemente más tranquila—. Y también buscaremos a alguien que le haga la limpia.

—Me parece un plan excelente —concluyó la Dra. Miller—. Están cuidando de Leo de todas las maneras posibles, y eso es lo que hace una familia. Regresen en una semana para un **chequeo**, o antes si notan algo preocupante.

Cuando la familia se fue, la Dra. Miller reflexionó. Había tratado el posible trauma físico, pero al reconocer y respetar la creencia del **susto**, también había tratado la ansiedad de la familia. Y a veces, curar la preocupación de la familia era el primer paso para curar al niño.

## Análisis de la Situación y Puntos Clave

**Nota Cultural y Lingüística:** El **susto** es un concepto fundamental en la medicina tradicional de muchas culturas hispanas. No es simplemente "estar asustado"; se considera una enfermedad real con síntomas como **apatía**, **insomnio**, **pérdida de apetito** y **depresión**. Ignorar o ridiculizar esta creencia puede romper la confianza con la familia. Un profesional de la salud debe abordarlo con respeto, como una parte válida de la experiencia del paciente.

## Vocabulario Médico Utilizado:

- **Examen físico (Physical exam)**: La evaluación estándar del paciente.
- **Pupilas (Pupils)**: Su reacción a la luz es un indicador neurológico clave.
- **Dolor / Hinchazón (Pain / Swelling)**: Signos básicos de lesión.
- **Reflejos (Reflexes)**: Parte del examen neurológico.
- **Concusión cerebral (Concussion)**: La principal preocupación médica a descartar.
- **Vómitos / Dolor de cabeza (Vomiting / Headache)**: Síntomas de alarma importantes en un traumatismo craneal.
- **Sala de emergencias (Emergency room)**: A dónde dirigirse si los síntomas empeoran.
- **Chequeo (Check-up)**: Cita de seguimiento.

## Estrategia de Comunicación:

1. **Validación y Respeto:** La Dra. Miller no discutió la validez del "susto". En su lugar, lo validó ("Gracias por compartir eso conmigo") y lo integró en su comprensión del problema.

2. **Tender Puentes, no Construir Muros:** En lugar de presentar la medicina y la creencia cultural como opuestas, encontró un terreno común. Usó el término "shock" o "trauma emocional" como un puente conceptual, permitiendo que ambas perspectivas coexistieran.

3. **Enfoque en el Objetivo Común:** El objetivo tanto de la doctora como de la familia era el mismo: que Leo se recuperara. Al centrarse en este objetivo compartido, pudo dar sus recomendaciones médicas sin que fueran percibidas como una imposición.

4. **Instrucciones Claras y Accionables:** Proporcionó una lista clara de **signos de alarma** (los "red flags" de una concusión). Esto le dio a la familia herramientas concretas para monitorear la salud física de Leo, cumpliendo con su deber como médica.

5. **Apoyo al Cuidado Integral:** Al aprobar el plan de la familia de buscar una "limpia" mientras seguían sus consejos médicos, apoyó un enfoque de cuidado holístico que atendía las necesidades físicas, emocionales y espirituales del niño y su familia.

# "¿ME ENTIENDE, M'IJA?": CONSTRUYENDO CONFIANZA CON UNA PACIENTE MAYOR Y SU FAMILIA

### Un caso de fisioterapia y la comunicación indirecta

David, un joven fisioterapeuta, revisaba el plan de tratamiento de Carmen Rivera, una mujer de 82 años a la que todos llamaban con respeto Doña Carmen. Hacía un mes que le habían operado de una **fractura de cadera**, y su progreso era más lento de lo esperado. En el papel, los ejercicios eran sencillos: levantamiento de piernas, flexiones de tobillo, pequeños pasos con el andador. En la práctica, cada sesión era una lucha.

Doña Carmen estaba sentada en una silla, con la mirada perdida. A su lado, como siempre, estaba su hija Luisa, una mujer de unos 50 años cuya energía contrastaba con la fragilidad de su madre.

—Buenos días, Doña Carmen, Luisa. ¿Cómo estamos hoy? —preguntó David con una sonrisa.

Luisa respondió de inmediato. —Está un poco adolorida hoy, David. Le duele la cadera por la mañana.

David asintió y se arrodilló para quedar a la altura de los ojos de Doña Carmen. —¿Del 1 al 10, Doña Carmen, qué tan fuerte es el **dolor**?

Doña Carmen miró a su hija, con una pregunta silenciosa en los ojos. Luisa intervino. —Dice que como un 4. No es tan malo, pero le molesta.

David notó la dinámica. Luisa, con la mejor de las intenciones, era la voz de su madre. Doña Carmen se había convertido en una espectadora de su propia recuperación. Esto tenía que cambiar.

—Luisa, ¿le parece bien si intento hablar directamente con su mamá por un momento? A veces me ayuda a entender mejor lo que siente —dijo David con amabilidad.

Luisa pareció sorprendida, pero asintió. —Claro, como usted diga.

David se acercó más a Doña Carmen, ignorando por un momento el plan de ejercicios. —¿Doña Carmen, aparte del dolor, hay algo que le preocupe de los ejercicios? ¿Algo que le dé miedo?

El cambio fue sutil, pero inmediato. Los ojos de Doña Carmen se encontraron con los de David por primera vez. Un temblor casi imperceptible recorrió sus labios antes de que susurrara: —Tengo miedo de caerme otra vez.

Luisa ahogó una exclamación. —¡Mamá! Pero si estamos aquí para ayudarla, no se va a caer.

Doña Carmen bajó la mirada, como si la hubieran regañado. Pero antes de hacerlo, lanzó una mirada fugaz y suplicante a su hija, una mirada que David interpretó claramente. Era un "¿Me entiende, m'ija?", un ruego silencioso por comprensión, no por soluciones.

David entendió que el problema no era la falta de fuerza, sino la falta de confianza. El trauma de la caída seguía presente.

—Gracias por decirme eso, Doña Carmen. Es lo más importante que he escuchado hoy —dijo David con sinceridad—. Su miedo es completamente normal. Y no vamos a hacer nada que la haga sentir insegura. Vamos a cambiar el plan.

Dejó el andador a un lado. —Hoy no vamos a caminar. Vamos a hacer **ejercicios** sentados. Quiero que sienta la fuerza en sus piernas de nuevo, pero sin ningún riesgo de caer.

Comenzó con un ejercicio simple. —Quiero que levante esta pierna, solo un poquito. Yo estaré aquí, con mi mano debajo de su rodilla. No la dejaré caer.

Al principio, el movimiento fue vacilante. Pero con la mano de David ofreciendo soporte y su voz tranquila repitiendo "Usted tiene el control", Doña Carmen comenzó a levantar la pierna un poco más alto. Después de varias repeticiones, una diminuta sonrisa se dibujó en su rostro.

—Ahora la otra pierna —indicó David—. Sienta cómo sus músculos trabajan. Esos son los músculos que la van a proteger de las caídas.

Trabajaron durante veinte minutos, solo con ejercicios sentados, enfocados en reconstruir no solo la fuerza muscular, sino la conexión y la confianza entre su mente y su cuerpo. Al final de la sesión, Doña Carmen respiraba un poco agitada, pero sus ojos brillaban de una forma que David no había visto antes.

Luisa había observado todo en silencio, con lágrimas en los ojos. Cuando David se levantó, ella le dijo en voz baja: —Gracias. No me había dado cuenta de cuánto miedo tenía. Solo quería que se mejorara rápido.

—La recuperación no es una carrera —respondió David—. Especialmente cuando hay miedo. Hoy dimos el paso más importante: Doña Carmen recuperó un poco de control.

Mientras se iban, David escuchó a Doña Carmen decirle a su hija en voz baja: —Hoy sí trabajé, m'ija. Hoy sí.

# Análisis de la Situación y Puntos Clave

**Nota Cultural y Lingüística:** La dinámica familiar es central. Los hijos adultos a menudo asumen el rol de cuidadores y portavoces, especialmente con padres mayores. Si bien es un acto de amor, puede marginar al paciente. El término **"Doña"** es una muestra de respeto fundamental al dirigirse a una mujer mayor. La frase de la paciente a su hija, **"¿Me entiende, m'ija?"**, no es literal, sino una expresión de una necesidad emocional profunda que no ha sido escuchada.

## Vocabulario Médico Utilizado:

- **Fisioterapia (Physical therapy)**: La especialidad del tratamiento.
- **Fractura de cadera (Hip fracture)**: El diagnóstico inicial.
- **Dolor (Pain)**: El síntoma principal que se debe evaluar constantemente.
- **Ejercicios (Exercises)**: El núcleo del plan de tratamiento de fisioterapia.
- **Andador (Walker)**: Equipo de asistencia común en rehabilitación.
- **Miedo a caer (Fear of falling)**: Un factor psicológico crucial en la rehabilitación geriátrica, que a menudo es una barrera más grande que la debilidad física.

## Estrategia de Comunicación:

1. **Identificar al Verdadero Comunicador:** David reconoció que, aunque Luisa hablaba, el mensaje importante estaba atrapado dentro de Doña Carmen. Pidió permiso para cambiar la dinámica de comunicación de manera respetuosa.

2. **Crear un Espacio Seguro:** Al arrodillarse, hacer contacto visual y hacer una pregunta abierta sobre el miedo, David cambió el enfoque de la tarea física a la experiencia emocional del paciente.

3. **Validar la Emoción:** La respuesta de David ("Su miedo es completamente normal") fue crucial. Validó el sentimiento de la paciente, reduciendo la vergüenza y abriendo la puerta a la confianza.

4. **Adaptar el Tratamiento al Paciente, no el Paciente al Tratamiento:** En lugar de forzar el plan existente, lo desechó y creó uno nuevo basado en la necesidad emocional de la paciente: la seguridad. Esto demuestra un cuidado verdaderamente centrado en el paciente.

5. **Empoderar al Paciente:** Al usar frases como "Usted tiene el control" y proporcionar apoyo físico tangible, le devolvió a Doña Carmen la sensación de autonomía sobre su propio cuerpo, que es el objetivo final de la rehabilitación.

# EL SILENCIO DE CARLOS

## Una consulta de salud mental y el estigma en la comunidad

Carlos, un hombre de 45 años con las manos curtidas por años de trabajo en la construcción, se sentó rígidamente en la silla del consultorio. No miró al Dr. Peña a los ojos. Había venido por un dolor de espalda persistente y dolores de cabeza que no se iban con nada.

—Llevo así como dos meses, doctor —dijo Carlos con voz monótona—. Me duele aquí, en la espalda baja. Y la cabeza, por las tardes, me va a estallar.

El Dr. Peña, un médico de atención primaria, asintió mientras tomaba notas. Realizó un examen físico exhaustivo, pero no encontró ninguna causa física evidente para el dolor de Carlos. Sus músculos no estaban particularmente tensos y no había signos de una hernia o lesión. Sin embargo, notó algo más: un agotamiento profundo en la mirada de Carlos, una falta de energía que iba más allá del simple cansancio físico.

—Carlos, su examen físico es normal. No veo una lesión en su espalda —dijo el Dr. Peña con cuidado—. A veces, cuando cargamos con mucho **estrés** o preocupaciones, el cuerpo encuentra una forma de decírnoslo. Puede manifestarse como dolor. ¿Ha estado bajo mucha presión últimamente?

Carlos se encogió de hombros, su mirada fija en un punto de la pared. —El trabajo es duro. Siempre lo ha sido.

El Dr. Peña decidió cambiar de táctica. Sabía que preguntar directamente sobre la **depresión** podría cerrar la conversación por completo. En la cultura de Carlos, muchos hombres veían la tristeza como una debilidad, no como una enfermedad.

—Entiendo. El cansancio del trabajo es una cosa, pero quiero preguntarle algo más. En las últimas semanas, ¿ha tenido problemas para dormir, incluso cuando está agotado? ¿O ha perdido el interés en hacer cosas que antes disfrutaba, como ver un partido de fútbol o pasar tiempo con la familia?

La pregunta sobre el **insomnio** pareció dar en el clavo. Carlos tragó saliva, y por primera vez, su fachada se resquebrajó un poco.

—No duermo bien —admitió en voz baja—. Me despierto a las tres de la mañana y ya no puedo volver a dormir. Y... no tengo ganas de nada.

Era la puerta que el Dr. Peña necesitaba. Este fenómeno, donde el sufrimiento emocional se expresa a través de síntomas físicos, se conoce como **somatización**. El dolor de espalda y los dolores de cabeza de Carlos no eran imaginarios; eran la manifestación física de su angustia.

—Gracias por decirme eso, Carlos. Lo que me describe es muy común. Cuando la mente está sobrecargada, el cuerpo paga el precio. El **insomnio**, la falta de ganas, el dolor... todo está conectado. No es una señal de que usted sea débil, al contrario, es una señal de que ha sido fuerte por demasiado tiempo.

El Dr. Peña hizo una pausa, dejando que las palabras calaran. —A esto le llamamos **depresión**. Es una condición médica, como la diabetes o la presión alta. Y tiene tratamiento.

Carlos permaneció en silencio, pero esta vez era un silencio pensativo, no defensivo.

—No estoy loco, doctor.

—Por supuesto que no —respondió el Dr. Peña con firmeza y calidez—. No tiene nada que ver con la locura. Tiene que ver con un desequilibrio químico en el cerebro, a menudo causado por el **estrés** crónico. Hay medicamentos que pueden ayudar, y también existe la **terapia** o **consejería**.

Vio la vacilación en el rostro de Carlos ante la palabra "terapia".

—Piénselo de esta manera —continuó—. La **consejería** es como hablar con un entrenador. Si quisiera fortalecer su cuerpo, iría a un gimnasio. Si quiere fortalecer su mente y encontrar herramientas para manejar el estrés, habla con un consejero. Es para aprender a manejar el peso que lleva encima.

El Dr. Peña no presionó más. Sabía que había plantado una semilla.

—No tiene que decidir nada hoy. Pero quiero que sepa que hay ayuda disponible. Me gustaría verlo de nuevo en dos semanas para ver cómo sigue. ¿Le parece bien?

Carlos finalmente levantó la vista y miró al doctor. Asintió lentamente. —Está bien, doctor. En dos semanas.

No fue una solución inmediata, pero fue un comienzo. El silencio se había roto, y en la lucha contra el estigma de la **salud mental**, ese primer paso era una victoria inmensa.

## Análisis de la Situación y Puntos Clave

**Nota Cultural y Lingüística:** El estigma en torno a la **salud mental** es una barrera significativa, especialmente para los hombres en muchas culturas latinas donde se valora la fortaleza y el estoicismo ("machismo"). Los pacientes pueden ser reacios a admitir sentimientos de tristeza o **ansiedad**. Es más probable que presenten síntomas físicos, un proceso conocido como **somatización**.

## Vocabulario Médico Utilizado:

- **Estrés (Stress)**: Un término neutral y socialmente aceptado que puede servir como punto de entrada para discutir la salud mental.

- **Insomnio (Insomnia)**: Un síntoma físico específico y común de la depresión y la ansiedad, más fácil de admitir para un paciente que los sentimientos emocionales.

- **Somatización (Somatization)**: El concepto clínico clave de la historia, donde la angustia psicológica se manifiesta como síntomas físicos.

- **Depresión (Depression)**: El Dr. Peña utiliza el término clínico, pero solo después de haber preparado el terreno y lo enmarca como una condición médica, no como un defecto de carácter.

- **Terapia / Consejería (Therapy / Counseling)**: Se presenta de una manera desestigmatizada, comparándola con un "entrenamiento" para manejar el estrés.

## Estrategia de Comunicación:

1. **Abordar lo Físico Primero:** El Dr. Peña validó la queja principal de Carlos (el dolor) realizando un examen físico completo. Esto construyó una base de confianza.

2. **Uso de Preguntas de Detección Indirectas:** En lugar de un cuestionario formal, integró las preguntas del PHQ-2 (pérdida de interés e insomnio) de forma natural en la conversación.

3. **Conectar Mente y Cuerpo:** La estrategia más importante fue explicar la conexión entre el estrés y el dolor físico. Esto permitió a Carlos entender sus síntomas sin sentirse avergonzado de su estado emocional.

4. **Normalizar y Desestigmatizar:** Frases como "es muy común" y "no es una señal de debilidad" fueron cruciales para reducir el estigma y la resistencia del paciente.

5. **Reencuadrar la Terapia:** La analogía de la consejería como un "entrenador para el estrés" es una excelente manera de hacer que el concepto de terapia sea más accesible y menos intimidante.

6. **Paciencia y Metas Realistas:** El Dr. Peña no esperaba que Carlos aceptara la terapia de inmediato. Su objetivo era abrir la puerta a la conversación y asegurar una cita de seguimiento, lo cual es un éxito en este tipo de consultas.

# "TENGO LA PRESIÓN ALTA... CREO"

## La confusión de un paciente con las instrucciones de la farmacia

La **farmacia** del barrio era el lugar donde el señor Benítez, un viudo de 74 años, se sentía más abrumado. Se acercó al mostrador con una bolsa de plástico llena de frascos de pastillas y se la entregó a Laura, la joven **farmacéutica**.

—Vengo a por mi **receta** —dijo en voz baja, casi avergonzado—. La del médico de la presión.

Laura tomó la nueva receta y luego miró la bolsa. Contenía al menos seis frascos diferentes, algunos casi vacíos, otros casi llenos. Reconoció la confusión en los ojos del señor Benítez; la veía todos los días.

—Por supuesto, señor Benítez. Permítame un momento —dijo con una sonrisa tranquilizadora—. ¿Le parece si nos sentamos un momento en la zona de consulta para revisar todo juntos? Así nos aseguramos de que tiene todo lo que necesita.

En la pequeña área privada, Laura vació la bolsa sobre la mesa. Era un rompecabezas de medicamentos: dos para la presión arterial de dos médicos diferentes, metformina para la diabetes, e insulina.

—Señor Benítez, veo que tiene varios medicamentos. ¿Me puede explicar cómo los está tomando?

El hombre suspiró. —Pues... la doctora del corazón me dio esta —dijo, señalando un frasco—. Y el médico de cabecera me dio esta otra para la presión. Tomo una por la mañana y otra por la noche, pero a veces se me olvida cuál es cuál. Y esta otra grande es para el **azúcar en la sangre**.

Laura entendió el problema de inmediato: polifarmacia sin una coordinación clara. Estaba tomando dos medicamentos similares, lo que podría causarle mareos o una bajada de presión peligrosa.

—Gracias por mostrarme todo. Vamos a organizarlo —dijo Laura, tomando un bloc de notas—. Empecemos por lo más importante. Esta pastilla, la metformina, es para controlar su nivel de **azúcar en la sangre**, o **glucosa**. La **dosis** correcta es fundamental. ¿Se mide el azúcar en casa?

El señor Benítez negó con la cabeza. —No me gusta pincharme el dedo.

—Lo entiendo. Hablemos de eso en un momento. Ahora, estas dos pastillas para la presión. Hacen casi lo mismo. Voy a llamar a sus médicos para aclarar cuál de las dos debemos continuar. No es seguro tomar ambas. Mientras tanto, solo tomará una de ellas.

Laura se tomó el tiempo para explicar el propósito de cada medicamento en un lenguaje sencillo, evitando hablar solo de los nombres de los fármacos y centrándose en su función.

—También es importante que sepa que, a veces, los medicamentos pueden tener **efectos secundarios** —continuó—. Por ejemplo, si se siente muy mareado después de tomar la pastilla de la presión, debe decírmelo. No es para asustarlo, sino para que esté informado.

Viendo que el señor Benítez seguía abrumado, Laura tuvo una idea. Sacó un **pastillero** semanal de un estante.

—Mire, esto nos va a ayudar. Es un **pastillero**. Tiene cajitas para cada día de la semana, y cada día está dividido en mañana, mediodía, tarde y noche.

Abrió los frascos y, con el señor Benítez observando, comenzó a colocar las pastillas correctas en los compartimentos correspondientes para toda la semana.

—¿Ve? Por la mañana, solo tiene que abrir la cajita del lunes que dice "MAÑANA" y tomarse lo que hay dentro. Ya no hay confusión.

Le escribió un horario simple en una hoja grande:

- ⊙ **MAÑANA (con el desayuno):** 1 pastilla para la presión, 1 pastilla para el azúcar.
- ⊙ NOCHE (con la cena): 1 pastilla para el azúcar.

—Esto es una maravilla —dijo el señor Benítez, mirando el pastillero con un alivio evidente. Era la primera vez que su complejo régimen de medicamentos parecía manejable—. Nadie se había tomado el tiempo de explicarme esto así.

—Ese es mi trabajo —respondió Laura—. No solo darle las medicinas, sino asegurarme de que entiende cómo usarlas para que le ayuden. La farmacia no es solo una tienda, es un lugar para cuidar su salud.

El señor Benítez se fue ese día no solo con sus medicinas, sino con un plan claro y la confianza de que podía manejar su salud.

## Análisis de la Situación y Puntos Clave

**Nota Profesional y Lingüística:** El rol del **farmacéutico** va mucho más allá de dispensar medicamentos. Son profesionales de la salud de primera línea, cruciales para la educación del paciente y la prevención de errores de medicación. La "revisión de la bolsa" (brown bag review) es una práctica excelente para identificar problemas de polifarmacia, duplicación de terapias y falta de adherencia.

## Vocabulario Médico Utilizado:

- **Farmacia / Farmacéutico(a) (Pharmacy / Pharmacist)**: El entorno y el profesional clave de esta historia.

- **Receta (Prescription)**: El documento que autoriza la dispensación de un medicamento.

- **Dosis (Dosage)**: La cantidad específica de un medicamento. Es fundamental que el paciente entienda la diferencia entre la dosis (ej. 500 mg) y la frecuencia (ej. dos veces al día).

- **Azúcar en la sangre / Glucosa (Blood sugar / Glucose)**: Términos intercambiables y esenciales para la educación sobre la diabetes.

- **Efectos secundarios (Side effects)**: Un concepto que debe explicarse de manera equilibrada para informar sin alarmar.

- **Pastillero (Pill organizer)**: Una herramienta práctica y visual que mejora enormemente la adherencia en pacientes con múltiples medicamentos.

## Estrategia de Comunicación:

1. **Crear un Entorno Privado:** Laura sacó al señor Benítez del mostrador público a un área de consulta. Esto es vital para discutir información de salud sensible y reduce la sensación de prisa y vergüenza del paciente.

2. **Enfoque en la Función, no en el Nombre:** En lugar de decir "tome el lisinopril y la metformina", Laura explicó lo que hacía cada pastilla ("esta es para la presión", "esta es para el azúcar"). Esto ayuda al paciente a entender el *porqué* de su tratamiento.

3. **Identificar y Resolver el Problema Central:** Laura no se limitó a dispensar la nueva receta. Identificó el problema de raíz (confusión y duplicación de terapia) y tomó una medida proactiva (llamar a los médicos) para resolverlo.

4. **Proporcionar Herramientas Prácticas:** La introducción del **pastillero** fue la intervención más efectiva. Transformó instrucciones abstractas y confusas en una acción física, simple y repetible.

5. **Empoderamiento del Paciente:** Al final de la consulta, el señor Benítez no solo tenía sus pastillas organizadas, sino que se sentía capaz de manejar su propio tratamiento. Laura le devolvió el control sobre su salud.

# "MI BEBÉ NO QUIERE COMER"

## Una consulta de lactancia con una madre primeriza

Sofía entró al consultorio de lactancia con pasos lentos y agotados. En sus brazos, acunaba a Mateo, su bebé de cinco días, que dormía plácidamente. Pero el rostro de Sofía estaba lleno de una ansiedad que contrastaba con la calma del recién nacido.

—Hola, Sofía. Soy Ana, la consultora de **lactancia**. Por favor, toma asiento. ¿Cómo te encuentras? —preguntó Ana, dirigiendo la primera pregunta a la madre, no al bebé.

Los ojos de Sofía se llenaron de lágrimas al instante. —No estoy bien. Siento que no sirvo para esto. Mi bebé no quiere comer.

Ana escuchó esa frase, "no quiere comer", y supo que era el comienzo de un misterio que debía resolver con delicadeza. Podía significar cualquier cosa, desde un problema real de succión hasta la simple ansiedad de una madre primeriza.

—Gracias por venir. Estás haciendo exactamente lo correcto al buscar ayuda —la tranquilizó Ana—. Antes de ver al bebé, quiero saber cómo estás tú. ¿Tienes dolor? ¿Has podido descansar algo?

Sofía negó con la cabeza. —Me duelen los pechos y estoy tan cansada que no puedo pensar.

—Eso es completamente normal los primeros días. Cuidar de un recién nacido es el trabajo más difícil del mundo. Ahora, hablemos de Mateo. En lugar de preguntarte si come o no, te haré una pregunta diferente: ¿cuántos **pañales mojados** ha tenido en las últimas 24 horas?

Sofía frunció el ceño, confundida. —¿Pañales? No sé... quizás cuatro o cinco.

—Perfecto. ¿Y pañales con popó?

—Uno hoy, era como amarillo con semillitas.

—¡Esas son excelentes noticias! —exclamó Ana con una sonrisa genuina—. Los pañales son la mejor manera de saber si un bebé está recibiendo suficiente leche. Y lo que me describes es completamente normal. Ahora, ¿te parece si me muestras cómo le das el pecho cuando se despierte?

Cuando Mateo comenzó a moverse, Ana guio a Sofía. —Vamos a hacer algo primero. Vamos a poner al bebé en contacto **piel con piel**. Quítale toda la ropita, déjalo solo con su pañal y ponlo directamente sobre tu pecho.

Mientras Sofía lo hacía, Ana explicó: —El contacto **piel con piel** es mágico. Ayuda a regular la temperatura del bebé, lo calma y despierta su instinto para comer.

Mateo, al sentir el calor de su madre, comenzó a buscar el pecho. Sofía lo guio, pero el bebé se quejó y se apartó después de unos segundos.

—¿Ves? No quiere —dijo Sofía, con la frustración a flor de piel.

—Veo algo diferente —dijo Ana con suavidad—. Veo un bebé que está intentando y una mamá que también lo intenta. Permíteme mostrarte algo.

Ana observó de cerca. —Tu bebé tiene un **agarre** un poco superficial. Eso significa que solo está succionando del pezón, y por eso se cansa y se frustra. Necesita tener una boca bien grande, como si fuera a morder una hamburguesa, para abarcar más pecho.

Con sus manos, le mostró a Sofía cómo sujetar su pecho y cómo acercar al bebé. —Espera a que abra la boca bien grande... ¡así! Ahora, acércalo rápido.

Guiada por Ana, Sofía lo intentó de nuevo. Esta vez, Mateo se prendió del pecho de una manera visiblemente más profunda. Su cuerpo se relajó y comenzó a succionar con un ritmo constante, con pausas en las que se podían oír pequeñas degluciones.

—Oh... —susurró Sofía, sintiendo la diferencia—. Ahora sí.

—Lo estás haciendo de maravilla —la animó Ana—. La **lactancia** no es algo que sale perfecto desde el primer día. Es un baile que tú y tu bebé están aprendiendo juntos. Requiere práctica y mucha paciencia.

Al final de la sesión, Ana le dio a Sofía una hoja simple para que apuntara los pañales y las tomas, no para obsesionarse, sino para tener la tranquilidad de que Mateo estaba bien.

—No estás sola en esto —le dijo Ana al despedirse—. Eres una madre increíble y estás haciendo un trabajo fantástico.

Sofía se fue del consultorio con los hombros un poco menos tensos y con una nueva confianza en su cuerpo y en su bebé. El misterio no estaba resuelto del todo, pero ahora tenía un mapa para navegarlo.

## Análisis de la Situación y Puntos Clave

**Nota Profesional y Lingüística:** La consulta de lactancia es un espacio emocionalmente vulnerable. El lenguaje debe ser de apoyo, sin juicios y empoderador. Frases como "no quiere comer" son una señal de angustia que requiere una investigación cuidadosa, no una aceptación literal. El enfoque en indicadores objetivos (pañales) en lugar de subjetivos (tiempo en el pecho) es una estrategia clínica clave.

## Vocabulario Médico Utilizado:

- **Lactancia (Breastfeeding/Lactation)**: El término general para el proceso. También se usa "amamantar".

- **Pañales mojados (Wet diapers)**: Un indicador clínico fundamental y fácil de medir para los padres sobre la ingesta del bebé.

- **Agarre (Latch)**: El término técnico para describir cómo el bebé se prende al pecho. Un buen o mal agarre es a menudo la clave del éxito o fracaso de la lactancia.

- **Piel con piel (Skin-to-skin)**: Una práctica basada en la evidencia que se recomienda para promover la lactancia, la regulación térmica y el vínculo afectivo.

## Estrategia de Comunicación:

1. **Enfocarse Primero en la Madre:** Ana comenzó preguntándole a Sofía cómo estaba ella. Esto valida los sentimientos de la madre y reconoce que su bienestar es inseparable del de su bebé.

2. **Usar Medidas Objetivas:** Cambiar la pregunta de "¿Está comiendo?" a "¿Cuántos pañales moja?" transforma una pregunta llena de ansiedad en una recolección de datos concretos y tranquilizadores.

3. **Observar en Lugar de Interrogar ("Show me"):** Pedirle a Sofía que le mostrara una toma le dio a Ana mucha más información que cualquier descripción verbal.

4. **Lenguaje Positivo y de Empoderamiento:** Ana utilizó frases como "Lo estás haciendo de maravilla" y "Eres una madre increíble". Este refuerzo positivo es vital para una madre agotada y ansiosa.

5. **Normalizar la Dificultad:** La analogía de la lactancia como "un baile que están aprendiendo juntos" normaliza la curva de aprendizaje y alivia la presión de tener que ser perfecta desde el principio.

# "ES QUE TRABAJO EN EL CAMPO"

## Un neumólogo investiga una tos crónica

El Dr. Ramírez, un neumólogo con una paciencia infinita, escuchaba atentamente a Javier, un hombre de 55 años cuyo rostro estaba surcado por el sol y el trabajo duro. La **tos** de Javier era seca, persistente y lo había acompañado durante casi un año.

—Empezó poco a poco, doctor. Ahora no me deja ni dormir —explicó Javier, interrumpiendo su propia frase con un acceso de tos.

—Lo entiendo. Vamos a llegar al fondo de esto —dijo el Dr. Ramírez—. En su **historia clínica** dice que usted no fuma. ¿Es correcto?

—Nunca he fumado un cigarrillo en mi vida.

—Excelente. ¿Y en su trabajo, está expuesto a mucho polvo, químicos o humo?

Javier se encogió de hombros. —Pues... **trabajo en el campo**. En la agricultura. Hay polvo, claro. Pero lo he hecho toda mi vida, nunca me había molestado.

El Dr. Ramírez sabía que "trabajo en el campo" podía significar muchas cosas. Necesitaba detalles.

—Cuénteme un poco más sobre su día a día. ¿Qué tipo de cultivos trabaja? ¿Usa algún tipo de pesticida o fertilizante?

—Trabajamos con maíz y soja. Y sí, usamos químicos para las plagas. Pero siempre me pongo una mascarilla de tela.

Una mascarilla de tela. El Dr. Ramírez anotó mentalmente que eso ofrecía una protección mínima.

—Gracias, eso es útil. Vamos a hacerle una **radiografía de tórax** para ver sus pulmones. Y también una prueba llamada **espirometría**.

Viendo la mirada de confusión de Javier, se apresuró a explicar. —La **espirometría** es muy sencilla. Usted va a soplar en un tubo con toda su fuerza. Nos ayuda a medir qué tan bien están funcionando sus pulmones, cuánta capacidad tienen. No duele nada.

Los resultados llegaron esa misma tarde. La radiografía mostraba un patrón difuso, como pequeñas sombras repartidas por los pulmones. La espirometría confirmó una función pulmonar reducida, un patrón restrictivo.

El Dr. Ramírez se sentó con Javier para explicarle los hallazgos.

—Javier, los exámenes muestran que sus pulmones tienen una inflamación crónica. Esto no es una infección ni cáncer. Creemos que es una reacción a algo que ha estado respirando durante mucho tiempo.

Javier lo miró sin comprender. —¿El polvo del campo?

—Posiblemente. Hay una condición llamada **neumonitis por hipersensibilidad**. Es una reacción alérgica del pulmón a partículas orgánicas, como el moho que puede crecer en el heno o el grano, o incluso a ciertos químicos agrícolas.

El doctor le mostró la radiografía. —Vea estas pequeñas manchas. Son la evidencia de la inflamación. Su cuerpo está reaccionando a algo en su ambiente de trabajo.

Javier parecía abrumado. —¿Y qué hago, doctor? Tengo que trabajar.

—Lo sé, y vamos a encontrar una solución. El primer paso es reducir la exposición. Necesita usar una mascarilla respiratoria adecuada, una N95 o superior, no una de tela. Y vamos a empezar un tratamiento con **corticosteroides**, unas pastillas que ayudarán a bajar la inflamación de sus pulmones.

Le recetó un tratamiento y le dio una orden para conseguir el equipo de protección adecuado.

—Esto es muy importante, Javier. Su salud depende de proteger sus pulmones. Quiero verlo en un mes para repetir la **espirometría** y ver cómo responde al tratamiento. Si evitamos lo que le está causando el daño y tratamos la inflamación, su **tos** debería mejorar mucho.

Javier asintió, esta vez con una expresión de entendimiento y determinación. Por primera vez en meses, sentía que su problema tenía un nombre y, lo más importante, una solución.

## Análisis de la Situación y Puntos Clave

**Nota Profesional y Lingüística:** La historia ocupacional es una parte crítica de la **historia clínica**, especialmente en neumología. Frases genéricas como **"trabajo en el campo"** son una señal para que el médico indague más a fondo. No todos los pacientes son conscientes de los riesgos específicos de su entorno laboral.

## Vocabulario Médico Utilizado:

- **Tos (Cough)**: El síntoma principal.
- **Radiografía de tórax (Chest X-ray)**: Una prueba de imagen fundamental para evaluar los pulmones.
- **Espirometría (Spirometry)**: La prueba clave para medir la función pulmonar. Es crucial explicarla en términos sencillos ("soplar en un tubo") para evitar la ansiedad del paciente.

- ⊙ **Neumonitis por hipersensibilidad (Hypersensitivity pneumonitis)**: El diagnóstico específico. Es un término complejo que el médico "traduce" a una explicación más simple ("reacción alérgica del pulmón").

- ⊙ **Corticosteroides (Corticosteroids)**: El tratamiento principal para reducir la inflamación en este tipo de condiciones.

## Estrategia de Comunicación:

1. **Indagación Detallada:** El Dr. Ramírez no se conformó con la respuesta inicial de Javier. Hizo preguntas específicas sobre el tipo de trabajo y la exposición, lo que le dio las pistas necesarias para el diagnóstico.

2. **Explicación Sencilla de Pruebas Complejas:** Su descripción de la **espirometría** fue tranquilizadora y fácil de entender, lo que aseguró la cooperación del paciente.

3. **Uso de Ayudas Visuales:** Mostrarle la radiografía al paciente y señalarle las anomalías lo involucró directamente en su diagnóstico, haciéndolo más tangible.

4. **Enfoque en Soluciones Prácticas:** El médico no solo dio un diagnóstico, sino que ofreció soluciones concretas y realistas (cambiar la mascarilla, iniciar tratamiento) que abordaban tanto la causa como los síntomas.

5. **Validación de las Circunstancias del Paciente:** Al decir "Lo sé, y vamos a encontrar una solución", el Dr. Ramírez reconoció la realidad económica de Javier ("Tengo que trabajar") en lugar de simplemente ordenarle que evitara la exposición, lo que habría sido poco realista y habría creado una barrera.

# LA DIETA DEL "ARROCITO Y POLLO"

## Adaptando las recomendaciones nutricionales a la cultura

María, una joven dietista, revisaba los resultados de laboratorio del señor Rojas, un hombre de 62 años con una sonrisa tan amplia como su amor por la buena comida. Su **colesterol** total estaba por las nubes, y los triglicéridos no se quedaban atrás.

—Buenos días, señor Rojas. Gracias por traer su diario de comidas —comenzó María, señalando la libreta que el paciente había dejado sobre la mesa.

—Ahí apunté todo, señorita. El desayuno con mis arepas, el almuerzo con mi buen sancocho, y por la noche, pues, un arrocito con pollo. No como mucho dulce —dijo él, casi a la defensiva.

María ojeó el diario. La dieta del señor Rojas era un delicioso mapa de la cocina tradicional de su país. También era rica en **grasas saturadas** y **carbohidratos** refinados. Sabía que decirle que dejara de comer todo lo que amaba sería una batalla perdida desde el principio.

—Se ve todo delicioso, señor Rojas. Entiendo perfectamente por qué le gusta tanto su comida —dijo ella con una sonrisa sincera. Esta validación inicial hizo que el señor Rojas se relajara visiblemente—. Mi trabajo no es quitarle lo que le gusta, sino encontrar maneras de hacerlo más saludable para su corazón.

Tomó una hoja y dibujó dos caminos. —Piense en el **colesterol** como el tráfico en una carretera. Hay un colesterol "malo" (LDL), que son como muchos carros creando un atasco en sus arterias. Y hay un colesterol "bueno" (HDL), que es como una grúa que limpia ese atasco.

El señor Rojas la miró, interesado en la analogía.

—Algunas de las comidas que nos encantan, como las frituras o la manteca, aumentan los carros malos. Otras, como el aguacate, el aceite de oliva y los frijoles, traen más grúas para limpiar. Queremos menos atascos y más grúas.

Señaló el diario de comidas. —¿El sancocho del almuerzo, lo prepara con mucha grasa?

—Bueno, un poquito, para que tenga sabor.

—Entiendo. ¿Y si en lugar de usar tanta grasa, le ponemos más verduras y hierbas para darle sabor? Y en lugar de tanto arroz blanco, podríamos probar con arroz integral, que tiene más **fibra**. La **fibra** es como una esponja que ayuda a atrapar el colesterol malo y a sacarlo del cuerpo.

María continuó, abordando cada comida con una sugerencia de modificación, no de eliminación.

—Las arepas del desayuno son deliciosas. ¿Qué tal si en lugar de comer tres, comemos una y media y la acompañamos con un poco de aguacate o huevo? Se sentirá igual de lleno, pero con más "grúas" para su colesterol. Y el pollo del "arrocito con pollo", ¿lo cocina con piel?

—Sí, claro, la piel es lo más rico.

—Lo sé —rió María—. Pero la piel tiene mucha grasa que crea "atascos". ¿Qué le parece si prueba cocinarlo sin piel y le pone más condimentos como ajo, cebolla y pimentón para que quede jugoso y con mucho sabor?

Al final de la consulta, el señor Rojas no se sentía privado, sino educado. María le había dado opciones, no órdenes.

—Vamos a empezar con algo pequeño —propuso María—. Esta semana, elija solo un cambio. ¿Quizás cocinar el pollo sin piel o añadir una porción extra de ensalada a su almuerzo?

El señor Rojas lo pensó. —Puedo intentar lo del pollo. Y lo del arroz integral... bueno, lo probaré.

—¡Excelente! —dijo María—. No se trata de una dieta estricta, señor Rojas. Se trata de hacer pequeños cambios inteligentes que pueda mantener para siempre. Su comida puede seguir siendo su comida, solo que un poco más amigable con su corazón.

Se fue con un plan de acción realista y, por primera vez, sin sentir que cuidar su salud significaba renunciar a su identidad.

## Análisis de la Situación y Puntos Clave

**Nota Cultural y Lingüística:** La comida es una parte fundamental de la identidad cultural y familiar. Las recomendaciones dietéticas que ignoran esto están destinadas al fracaso. Un enfoque exitoso no prohíbe, sino que adapta. El uso de analogías simples (el tráfico, las grúas, la esponja) es una herramienta de comunicación muy poderosa para explicar conceptos abstractos.

### Vocabulario Médico Utilizado:

- ⊙ **Colesterol (Cholesterol)**: El concepto central de la consulta. Es vital diferenciar entre el "bueno" (HDL) y el "malo" (LDL) en términos que el paciente pueda entender.

- ⊙ **Grasas saturadas (Saturated fats)**: El tipo de grasa que se debe limitar. En lugar de usar el término técnico, se puede hablar de "grasa de la piel del pollo" o "manteca".

- ⊙ **Carbohidratos (Carbohydrates)**: Se aborda de manera práctica al hablar de "arroz blanco" versus "arroz integral".

- ⊙ **Fibra (Fiber)**: Se explica su función con una analogía fácil de recordar ("es como una esponja").

- ⊙ **Porciones (Portions)**: Un concepto clave en el control de la dieta, que se introduce de manera sutil ("en lugar de tres arepas, una y media").

## Estrategia de Comunicación:

1. **Validar Antes de Aconsejar:** María comenzó validando la cultura y el gusto del paciente por su comida. Esto creó una alianza inmediata y demostró respeto.

2. **Modificación, no Eliminación:** La estrategia central fue sugerir "intercambios" saludables en lugar de prohibir alimentos. Esto reduce la resistencia y hace que el plan sea sostenible a largo plazo.

3. **Uso de Analogías Claras:** Las metáforas del tráfico y la esponja tradujeron la bioquímica del colesterol y la fibra en imágenes cotidianas, facilitando la comprensión y la retención.

4. **Enfoque en Metas Pequeñas y Realistas:** Al pedirle al paciente que eligiera solo un cambio para empezar, María hizo que la tarea pareciera manejable y no abrumadora, aumentando las probabilidades de éxito.

5. **Lenguaje Colaborativo:** Usó frases como "¿Qué le parece si...?" y "Podríamos probar...", que invitan a la colaboración en lugar de imponer una directiva. Esto respeta la autonomía del paciente y lo convierte en socio de su propio plan de salud.

# "NO QUIERO QUE ME PINCHEN MÁS"

## Manejando el miedo a las agujas en un paciente con diabetes tipo 1

Daniela, una enfermera educadora en diabetes, sabía que esta sería la consulta más difícil del día. Frente a ella estaba Leo, un chico de 15 años diagnosticado con **diabetes tipo 1** la semana anterior. Su rostro estaba cerrado en una máscara de rebeldía adolescente, pero sus manos, apretadas en puños sobre sus rodillas, delataban su miedo. A su lado, su madre, Marta, parecía al borde de las lágrimas.

—Leo, hoy vamos a practicar cómo ponerte la **inyección** de **insulina** tú solo. Es un paso muy importante para que puedas volver a tu vida normal, a jugar al fútbol —comenzó Daniela con una voz suave y alentadora.

Colocó sobre la mesa una pluma de insulina de práctica y una pequeña almohadilla que simulaba la piel.

La reacción de Leo fue inmediata y visceral. Se echó hacia atrás en su silla. —No. No quiero que me pinchen más. En el hospital ya fue suficiente.

Marta intervino, su voz teñida de desesperación. —Leo, por favor. Tienes que hacerlo. Es por tu bien.

—¡Tú no lo entiendes! ¡A ti no te están clavando una **aguja** cuatro veces al día! —replicó él, su voz quebrándose.

Daniela levantó una mano con calma. —Marta, ¿le importaría darnos a Leo y a mí unos minutos a solas? Creo que nos vendría bien hablar un poco.

Marta asintió, agradecida, y salió del consultorio. Daniela se giró hacia Leo, pero no se acercó a la mesa de práctica. Simplemente se sentó frente a él.

—Tienes toda la razón —dijo ella, sorprendiendo a Leo—. Que te pinchen apesta. Y tienes derecho a odiarlo.

Leo la miró, desconfiado. No esperaba esa respuesta.

—Lo que sentiste en el hospital fue muy duro. Las agujas para sacar sangre son más grandes, y todo es nuevo y aterrador. Pero la **insulina** es diferente. ¿Me permites mostrarte algo? No voy a pincharte. Solo quiero mostrarte.

Leo asintió con cautela. Daniela tomó la pluma de insulina y quitó el capuchón, revelando una aguja diminuta, casi invisible.

—Mira qué pequeña es. Es más fina que un cabello. La mayoría de la gente se sorprende de que apenas se siente. Pero no tienes que creerme. Tienes que sentirlo tú mismo cuando estés listo. El objetivo de hoy no es que te inyectes. El objetivo de hoy es que tú tomes el control.

Dejó la pluma en las manos de Leo. —Este aparato te da el poder. La diabetes te quitó algo, el poder de tu cuerpo para usar la energía. Esto te lo devuelve.

Luego, le explicó de una manera que un chico de 15 años podría entender. —Piensa en la comida como la gasolina para un coche de carreras. Tu cuerpo es el coche. Pero ahora mismo, la puerta del depósito de gasolina está cerrada con llave. La **insulina** es la única llave que puede abrirla. Sin ella, tienes toda la gasolina del mundo, pero el motor no puede usarla. Por eso te sentías tan cansado antes del diagnóstico.

Leo miraba la pluma en su mano. La analogía del coche de carreras pareció resonar en él.

—¿Quieres volver a jugar al fútbol? —preguntó Daniela.

—Sí.

—Entonces necesitas gasolina en el motor. Necesitas esta llave. Y la buena noticia es que tú eres el único que puede usarla. Tú decides cuándo, tú decides dónde. Es tu poder, no el de la diabetes. ¿Quieres probar cómo se siente usarla en esta almohadilla? Solo el movimiento.

Leo dudó, pero finalmente tomó la almohadilla. Daniela guio sus manos para mostrarle el ángulo correcto, cómo presionar el botón. Lo hizo una, dos, tres veces. Un simple clic. Sin aguja, sin dolor. Solo control.

—Bien hecho —dijo Daniela—. Ahora, si te sientes capaz, podemos ponerle la aguja y probarlo en la almohadilla.

Leo respiró hondo y asintió. Realizó la **inyección** en la almohadilla de práctica. Miró la pequeña gota de solución salina sobre la superficie. Era él quien lo había hecho.

—No fue tan malo —murmuró.

—Nunca lo es tanto como nuestra mente nos dice —respondió Daniela con una sonrisa—. El miedo es el verdadero pinchazo. Lo que acabas de hacer se llama **autocontrol**. Y es el primer paso para ser el jefe de tu diabetes, y no al revés.

No se inyectó él mismo ese día. Pero cuando su madre volvió a entrar, Leo sostenía la pluma de insulina en su mano, no como un arma que le atacaba, sino como una herramienta que le pertenecía.

## Análisis de la Situación y Puntos Clave

**Nota Profesional y Lingüística:** El diagnóstico de una enfermedad crónica en un adolescente presenta desafíos únicos. La necesidad de independencia choca con la dependencia del tratamiento. El lenguaje debe ser de empoderamiento, no de imposición. El miedo a las agujas (belonefobia) es real y debe ser tratado con técnicas de desensibilización y manejo del control.

### Vocabulario Médico Utilizado:

- **Diabetes tipo 1 (Type 1 diabetes)**: El diagnóstico. Es crucial diferenciarlo del tipo 2, ya que el tratamiento con insulina es innegociable.
- **Insulina (Insulin)**: La hormona y el medicamento central de la historia.
- **Inyección (Injection)**: El acto de administrar el medicamento.
- **Aguja (Needle)**: El objeto del miedo del paciente. Desmitificar su tamaño y la sensación que produce es una estrategia clave.
- **Autocontrol (Self-management)**: El objetivo final de la educación en diabetes. Se refiere a la capacidad del paciente para manejar su propia condición.

### Estrategia de Comunicación:

1. **Validar la Emoción, no Descartarla:** La primera y más importante acción de Daniela fue validar el enojo y el miedo de Leo ("Tienes toda la razón. Que te pinchen apesta"). Esto desarmó la resistencia del paciente y construyó una alianza.

2. **Crear un Espacio Privado y Seguro:** Pedirle a la madre que saliera fue esencial. Permitió una conversación honesta sin la presión o la angustia parental, dándole a Leo la oportunidad de ser vulnerable.

3. **Cambiar el Paradigma del Control:** Daniela reformuló la situación. La inyección no era algo que "le hacían a él", sino una herramienta que "él usaba". Poner la pluma en su mano fue un acto simbólico de transferirle el poder.

4. **Uso de Analogías Relevantes:** La metáfora de la "llave para el depósito de gasolina" conectó el tratamiento directamente con el objetivo personal de Leo (jugar al fútbol). Esto le dio al tratamiento un propósito significativo para él, más allá de la simple supervivencia.

5. **Desensibilización Gradual:** El proceso de practicar primero el movimiento sin aguja, y luego en una almohadilla, es una técnica de desensibilización conductual. Reduce la ansiedad al dividir una tarea abrumadora en pasos pequeños y manejables.

6. **Establecer Metas Realistas:** Daniela reconoció que el éxito de la sesión no era necesariamente que Leo se inyectara, sino que comenzara a superar su miedo y aceptara el concepto de **autocontrol**. Esto evita la presión y celebra el progreso, por pequeño que sea.

# "¿Y ESO LO CUBRE EL SEGURO?"

## Navegando el sistema de salud con un paciente recién llegado

La oficina del cirujano era impecable y moderna, pero para la familia Reyes, se sentía como un laberinto intimidante. Javier, el padre, necesitaba una cirugía para reparar una hernia inguinal que le causaba un dolor constante. Su hija, Sofía, de 22 años, lo acompañaba, actuando como traductora y defensora, con el peso del mundo sobre sus jóvenes hombros.

Después de hablar con el cirujano, fueron dirigidos a la oficina de Ana, la coordinadora de servicios para pacientes. Ana, una mujer cálida y bilingüe, notó de inmediato la tensión en sus rostros.

—Hola, Javier, Sofía. Soy Ana. Mi trabajo es ayudarles a entender los próximos pasos, especialmente lo que tiene que ver con el pago y el **seguro** —dijo en un español claro y acogedor.

Sofía soltó un suspiro de alivio al escuchar su idioma. —Gracias. Estamos muy confundidos. El doctor dice que mi papá necesita la operación, pero no tenemos idea de cuánto va a costar. Acabamos de llegar a este país y el sistema es muy complicado. ¿Y eso lo cubre el **seguro**?

Era la pregunta que Ana escuchaba todos los días, cargada de miedo a una deuda impagable.

—Esa es la pregunta más importante, y vamos a resolverla juntos —respondió Ana, invitándolos a sentarse—. Primero, quiero que sepan que es normal sentirse así. Vamos a ir paso a paso.

Tomó una hoja de papel. —Lo primero que haremos es pedir una **autorización previa** a su compañía de seguros. Esto significa que nosotros, la oficina del doctor, les enviamos toda la información médica de su papá y les pedimos permiso para hacer la cirugía. No programaremos nada hasta que el seguro nos dé el visto bueno.

Javier, que había estado en silencio, preguntó con voz preocupada: —¿Y si dicen que no?

—Es una buena pregunta. Si dicen que no, tenemos derecho a apelar. Pero para una hernia como la suya, que le causa dolor, es muy probable que la aprueben. Es una cirugía médicamente necesaria.

Luego, Ana abordó el tema del costo. —Ahora, hablemos de lo que ustedes podrían tener que pagar. Su plan de **seguro** tiene algo que se llama **deducible**.

Viendo sus miradas en blanco, simplificó la explicación. —Imaginen que el **deducible** es como una cantidad que ustedes deben pagar primero de su bolsillo cada año. Digamos que su deducible es de mil dólares. Ustedes pagan los primeros mil dólares de sus gastos médicos, y después de eso, el seguro empieza a pagar un porcentaje alto, como el 80% o 90% del resto.

Sofía lo procesó. —¿Así que tenemos que saber si ya hemos pagado algo de ese deducible este año?

—Exactamente —dijo Ana, impresionada por la rapidez de Sofía—. Yo puedo ayudarles a verificar eso con su seguro. También está el **copago**, que es una cantidad fija que pagan por cada consulta, pero eso es diferente del costo de la cirugía.

Les mostró un formulario. —Una vez que tengamos la autorización, les daremos un estimado de los costos. Incluirá los honorarios del cirujano, del anestesiólogo y del hospital. No será una sorpresa.

Ana también les habló de los recursos disponibles. —Si el costo que les corresponde pagar es demasiado alto, no se asusten. El hospital tiene programas de asistencia financiera y podemos establecer un plan de pagos sin intereses. No están solos en esto. Hay un **trabajador social** en el hospital que puede guiarles.

Al final de la reunión de treinta minutos, la nube de pánico que rodeaba a la familia Reyes se había disipado. El costo no había desaparecido, pero el miedo a lo desconocido sí. Tenían un plan, una secuencia de pasos lógicos y, lo más importante, una aliada.

—Gracias, de verdad —dijo Sofía, con una gratitud genuina—. Ahora entiendo.

—Para eso estoy aquí —respondió Ana—. Para que ustedes puedan concentrarse en lo más importante: que su papá se recupere. Nosotros nos encargamos del papeleo.

Javier le estrechó la mano a Ana, y aunque no dijo mucho, su apretón de manos y la tranquilidad en su mirada lo dijeron todo. Salieron de la oficina no con todas las respuestas, pero sí con la certeza de que podían navegar el laberinto.

## Análisis de la Situación y Puntos Clave

**Nota Profesional y Lingüística:** Navegar el sistema de salud de EE. UU. es un desafío incluso para los nativos. Para los recién llegados, la terminología del **seguro** es una barrera inmensa. Profesionales como coordinadores de pacientes, navegadores o **trabajadores sociales** son vitales. Su rol es traducir un sistema complejo a un lenguaje humano y comprensible.

### Vocabulario Médico Utilizado:

- ⊙ **Seguro (Insurance)**: El término general para la cobertura médica.
- ⊙ **Cobertura (Coverage)**: Describe qué servicios y en qué medida están pagados por el plan de seguro.

- **Autorización previa (Prior authorization)**: Un paso administrativo crucial que el personal médico debe gestionar antes de muchos procedimientos para garantizar el pago del seguro.

- **Deducible (Deductible)**: Uno de los conceptos más confusos para los pacientes. La analogía de "pagar primero una cantidad" antes de que el seguro ayude es una forma efectiva de explicarlo.

- **Copago (Copay)**: Un costo más simple y directo, pero que debe diferenciarse del deducible y del coseguro.

- **Trabajador(a) social (Social worker)**: Un recurso clave para pacientes que enfrentan barreras socioeconómicas, incluyendo la dificultad para pagar la atención médica.

## Estrategia de Comunicación:

1. **Validar la Ansiedad:** Ana comenzó reconociendo que la confusión y el miedo del paciente eran normales. Esto inmediatamente bajó las defensas de la familia y creó una relación de confianza.

2. **Dividir el Proceso en Pasos:** En lugar de abrumarlos con toda la información a la vez, dividió el proceso en una secuencia lógica: primero la autorización, luego el estimado de costos, y finalmente los recursos de ayuda.

3. **Uso de Lenguaje Sencillo y Analogías:** Explicó los términos técnicos del seguro (deducible) usando un lenguaje llano y analogías fáciles de entender, en lugar de definiciones formales.

4. **Proactividad y Definición de Roles:** Dejó claro qué haría la oficina ("nosotros pediremos la autorización") y qué podía esperar la familia. Esto les dio seguridad al saber que no tenían que hacer el trabajo pesado ellos solos.

5. **Enfoque en Soluciones, no solo en Problemas:** Ana no solo explicó los costos potenciales, sino que inmediatamente ofreció soluciones (planes de pago, asistencia financiera), lo que transformó una conversación aterradora en una de empoderamiento y esperanza.

6. **Crear un Sentido de Equipo:** Con frases como "vamos a resolverlo juntos" y "no están solos", Ana se posicionó como una aliada, cambiando la dinámica de "el sistema contra nosotros" a "nosotros juntos navegando el sistema".

# "DICE QUE LE DUELE LA PANZA"

### Diferenciando el dolor abdominal en un niño que no habla

La Dra. Chen, una médica de urgencias pediátricas, se acercó a la camilla donde estaba sentado Mateo, un niño de 7 años con el rostro pálido y surcado de lágrimas silenciosas. Se abrazaba el abdomen con fuerza. A su lado, sus padres, Luis y Elena, la miraban con una mezcla de miedo y agotamiento.

—Hola, soy la Dra. Chen. ¿Qué le pasa a Mateo? —preguntó ella, dirigiendo una sonrisa tranquilizadora al niño, que apenas la miró.

—Empezó anoche, doctora —dijo Luis, el padre—. Dice que le duele la **panza**. Tuvo un poco de **fiebre** y vomitó una vez después de la cena. Pensamos que era algo que había comido, pero hoy el dolor es peor.

La palabra **"panza"** era el término más común y vago que la Dra. Chen escuchaba en su turno. Podía ser cualquier cosa: gases, una indigestión, un virus estomacal o, su principal sospecha, **apendicitis**. La clave era diferenciar.

—Mateo, campeón, ¿puedes señalarme con un dedo exactamente dónde te duele más? —preguntó la doctora.

Mateo, entre sollozos, movió su mano vagamente sobre todo el área del ombligo. No era específico.

—Entiendo. A veces el dolor se mueve por todas partes —dijo la Dra. Chen con paciencia. Sabía que interrogar a un niño asustado y con dolor no la llevaría a ninguna parte. Tenía que observar.

—Voy a escucharte la barriga, ¿vale? Mi estetoscopio puede que esté un poco frío.

Mientras escuchaba, notó que los sonidos intestinales estaban disminuidos. Luego, se preparó para el paso más importante: **palpar** el abdomen.

—Muy bien, Mateo. Ahora vamos a jugar un juego. Voy a tocar tu barriga muy suavemente. Tú me dices "alto" cuando sientas mi mano en el lugar que más te duele.

Comenzó por el lado izquierdo, lejos del área de sospecha. Mateo apenas reaccionó. Luego se movió hacia arriba, y después hacia el lado derecho. Al presionar suavemente en el cuadrante inferior derecho, el cuerpo de Mateo se tensó y un gemido escapó de sus labios.

—¿Ahí? —preguntó ella.

Mateo asintió, con los ojos llenos de lágrimas.

La Dra. Chen tenía un signo clínico, pero necesitaba confirmarlo. La sensibilidad de rebote era difícil de evaluar en un niño porque el movimiento rápido podía asustarlo. Así que usó una técnica diferente.

—Luis —dijo, dirigiéndose al padre—, voy a pedirle que me ayude. Ponga su mano aquí, sobre la mía. Ahora, presione suavemente, como yo.

Luis lo hizo.

—Ahora, cuando yo le diga, quite su mano rápido.

—¡Ahora!

Luis levantó la mano. El cambio súbito de presión hizo que Mateo gritara de dolor, un llanto agudo y localizado. Era el signo que la Dra. Chen buscaba.

Se enderezó y miró a los padres. Su tono cambió de juguetón a seriamente compasivo.

—Gracias por traerlo. Creo que sé lo que tiene. Los signos que muestra Mateo son muy consistentes con una **apendicitis**.

Elena, la madre, se llevó una mano a la boca. —¿El apéndice? ¿Está segura?

—Los síntomas físicos apuntan a eso —explicó la Dra. Chen—. El apéndice es una pequeña bolsita conectada al intestino. Cuando se inflama, causa el tipo de dolor que Mateo tiene. Para estar completamente seguros, vamos a hacer un **ultrasonido**. Es como una fotografía del interior de su barriga que se hace con un gel y un aparatito. No duele nada.

El **ultrasonido** confirmó el diagnóstico: un apéndice inflamado y lleno de líquido. La Dra. Chen volvió con los padres.

—El ultrasonido lo confirma. Mateo necesita una **cirugía** para quitarle el apéndice. Es una operación muy común y segura. El cirujano vendrá a hablar con ustedes en unos minutos para explicarles todo el proceso.

Luis y Elena estaban asustados, pero la claridad y la confianza de la Dra. Chen los había anclado.

—Hicieron lo correcto al venir de inmediato —les dijo—. Confíen en su instinto de padres. Ustedes son los mejores expertos en su hijo.

Mientras se llevaban a Mateo para prepararlo para la **cirugía**, la Dra. Chen reflexionó sobre el delicado arte de la pediatría. A veces, el diagnóstico no se encontraba en las palabras del paciente, sino en el silencio, en un gemido, o en la tensión de un pequeño cuerpo que decía todo lo que necesitaba saber.

## Análisis de la Situación y Puntos Clave

**Nota Profesional y Lingüística:** En pediatría, el historial clínico a menudo lo proporcionan los padres, pero el examen físico depende de la habilidad del médico para interpretar signos no verbales. El uso de términos coloquiales como **"panza"** es común, y el profesional debe traducirlo a un contexto clínico.

## Vocabulario Médico Utilizado:

- ⊙ **Panza (Tummy/Belly)**: Término coloquial para abdomen. Es importante usarlo para conectar con la familia, pero pensar en términos anatómicos precisos (cuadrantes abdominales).

- ⊙ **Fiebre / Vómito (Fever / Vomiting)**: Síntomas clásicos que acompañan a muchas condiciones pediátricas, incluyendo la apendicitis.

- ⊙ **Apendicitis (Appendicitis)**: El diagnóstico central de la historia.

- ⊙ **Palpar (To palpate)**: El verbo clave para el examen físico del abdomen.

- ⊙ **Ultrasonido (Ultrasound)**: La prueba de imagen de elección en niños para evitar la radiación, especialmente en casos de sospecha de apendicitis.

- ⊙ **Cirugía (Surgery)**: El tratamiento definitivo para la apendicitis.

## Estrategia de Comunicación:

1. **Involucrar al Niño de Forma Lúdica:** La Dra. Chen convirtió el examen en un "juego" para reducir el miedo de Mateo y obtener una respuesta más fiable.

2. **Confiar en los Signos, no en las Palabras:** Dado que Mateo no podía localizar el dolor, la doctora se basó en signos clínicos objetivos (tensión muscular, reacción a la palpación) para guiar su diagnóstico.

3. **Involucrar a los Padres en el Examen:** Pedirle al padre que participara en la prueba de sensibilidad de rebote fue una estrategia brillante. Hizo que el signo fuera evidente para los padres y menos aterrador para el niño que si lo hiciera un extraño.

4. **Explicación Clara y Directa:** Una vez que tuvo una fuerte sospecha, la Dra. Chen fue directa con los padres, pero usó un lenguaje sencillo para explicar qué era la apendicitis y por qué el ultrasonido era necesario.

5. **Manejo de la Ansiedad Parental:** Reconoció el miedo de los padres y los tranquilizó, no con falsas promesas, sino con un plan de acción claro y seguro (ultrasonido, consulta con el cirujano).

6. **Empoderamiento de los Padres:** La frase final, "Confíen en su instinto de padres", validó su decisión de buscar ayuda y reforzó su rol como cuidadores competentes, fortaleciendo la alianza terapéutica.

# "EL PAPELITO LO DICE TODO"

## La importancia de la comunicación verbal más allá de los resultados de laboratorio

El Dr. Fuentes, un médico internista, tenía frente a él a Ricardo, un hombre de 48 años, contador de profesión, que vivía su vida a través de los números y los hechos concretos. Ricardo había acudido a la consulta por un cansancio extremo, aumento de peso y una sensación de frío que no lo abandonaba.

—Aquí están los **resultados de laboratorio** que me pidió, doctor —dijo Ricardo, deslizando una hoja de papel sobre el escritorio con la seguridad de quien entrega una prueba irrefutable—. Como puede ver, casi todo está en el rango normal.

El Dr. Fuentes tomó el informe. Ricardo tenía razón, sus niveles de colesterol y glucosa estaban bien. Pero el doctor se fijó en un valor específico: la TSH, la hormona estimulante de la **tiroides**. Estaba en 6.5 mU/L, por encima del rango de referencia del laboratorio, que marcaba un límite superior de 4.5.

—Gracias por traerlos, Ricardo. Efectivamente, la mayoría de sus valores están bien, pero hay uno que nos da la pista que necesitábamos —dijo el Dr. Fuentes, señalando el resultado de la TSH—. Este número de aquí está un poco elevado.

Ricardo frunció el ceño. —¿Un poco? Pero no está marcado en rojo ni nada. No parece importante.

Ahí estaba el desafío. Para Ricardo, si no era un número dramáticamente fuera de rango, no era un problema. El "papelito", como él lo veía, no gritaba "peligro".

—Entiendo su punto de vista —explicó el Dr. Fuentes con paciencia—. Pero en medicina, no solo miramos los números, sino lo que significan en el contexto de sus síntomas. La TSH es una **hormona** que funciona como un mensajero. Su cerebro la envía para pedirle a su glándula **tiroides**, que está aquí en el cuello, que trabaje.

Hizo una pausa para asegurarse de que Ricardo lo seguía. —Si su nivel de TSH está alto, es como si su cerebro estuviera gritándole a la tiroides: "¡Oye, trabaja más duro!". Y le grita porque la tiroides se ha vuelto un poco perezosa y no está produciendo suficientes hormonas por sí misma.

Ricardo seguía escéptico. —Pero es una diferencia pequeña.

—Es una diferencia pequeña en el papel, pero grande para su cuerpo. La tiroides es como el motor que regula la energía de todo su cuerpo. Si funciona lento, usted se siente lento. Por eso el cansancio, el frío, el aumento de peso. Sus síntomas encajan perfectamente con lo que este número nos dice. Esta condición se llama **hipotiroidismo subclínico**.

El Dr. Fuentes se reclinó en su silla. —Piénselo como el aceite del motor de su coche. Si el nivel está un poco bajo, el coche sigue andando, pero el motor se está forzando y, con el tiempo, se desgastará. Este "papelito" no lo dice todo. Me dice *qué* está pasando, pero sus síntomas me dicen *cómo* le está afectando. La combinación de ambos nos da el diagnóstico completo.

Ricardo procesó la información. La analogía del coche, un sistema lógico que él entendía, pareció conectar los puntos.

—Entonces, ¿necesito tratamiento?

—Sí. Iniciaremos un tratamiento con una dosis muy baja de la hormona tiroidea que su cuerpo no está produciendo en cantidad suficiente. Es una pastilla pequeña que tomará cada mañana. Debería empezar a sentirse con más energía en unas pocas semanas. En seis semanas, repetiremos el **análisis de sangre** para asegurarnos de que la dosis es la correcta.

El Dr. Fuentes le entregó la receta. —El tratamiento no se basa solo en este número, Ricardo. Se basa en usted. El objetivo no es solo que sus números se vean bien en el papel, sino que usted se sienta bien en su vida diaria.

Por primera vez en la consulta, Ricardo no miró el informe de laboratorio, sino directamente al doctor. —Entiendo. Gracias por explicármelo así, doctor.

Había llegado confiando solo en el "papelito", pero se fue confiando en la persona que sabía interpretarlo.

## Análisis de la Situación y Puntos Clave

**Nota Profesional y Lingüística:** En la era de la información, muchos pacientes tienen acceso a sus **resultados de laboratorio** antes de hablar con su médico. Pueden llegar a conclusiones erróneas, ya sea por alarma excesiva o, como en este caso, por minimizar hallazgos clínicamente significativos. El rol del médico es traducir los datos en un relato coherente que conecte con la experiencia del paciente.

### Vocabulario Médico Utilizado:

- **Resultados de laboratorio (Lab results)**: El documento central de la historia.
- **Tiroides (Thyroid)**: La glándula implicada en el diagnóstico.
- **Hormonas (Hormones)**: El concepto bioquímico clave, explicado como "mensajeros".
- **Hipotiroidismo (Hypothyroidism)**: El diagnóstico específico. El Dr. Fuentes añade el matiz de "subclínico" para ser preciso, pero lo explica en términos funcionales.

○ **Análisis de sangre (Blood test)**: El procedimiento utilizado para obtener los resultados.

## Estrategia de Comunicación:

1. **Validar la Observación del Paciente:** El Dr. Fuentes no contradijo a Ricardo. Estuvo de acuerdo en que la mayoría de los valores eran normales, validando la lectura inicial del paciente antes de introducir la excepción.

2. **Uso de Analogías Efectivas:** La metáfora del cerebro "gritándole" a la tiroides y la del "aceite del motor" fueron cruciales. Tradujeron un concepto endocrinológico complejo a un lenguaje cotidiano y lógico que un contador podía apreciar.

3. **Conectar los Datos con los Síntomas:** La estrategia más importante fue vincular directamente el número elevado de TSH con los síntomas específicos de Ricardo (cansancio, frío). Esto demostró que el "papelito" y su experiencia personal contaban la misma historia.

4. **Enfatizar el Contexto Clínico:** El Dr. Fuentes enseñó una lección fundamental de la medicina: un dato de laboratorio aislado tiene un valor limitado. Su verdadero significado proviene del contexto clínico del paciente.

5. **Enfocar el Tratamiento en el Bienestar del Paciente:** Al final, el objetivo del tratamiento no era "arreglar un número", sino "hacer que usted se sienta bien". Esto reorientó la meta de la consulta desde los datos abstractos hacia la calidad de vida del paciente, que es el fin último de la medicina.

# "VENGO POR UN CHEQUEO GENERAL"

## Descubriendo un problema subyacente durante un examen de rutina

Laura, una mujer de 34 años, se sentó en la camilla del consultorio de la Dra. Soto. Su sonrisa era amable, pero no llegaba a sus ojos, que parecían cansados.

—Hola, Laura. ¿En qué te puedo ayudar hoy? —preguntó la Dra. Soto, usando el tono cercano que reservaba para sus pacientes habituales.

—Solo vengo por un **chequeo general**, doctora. Hacía tiempo que no me hacía uno. Todo está bien, solo un poco de estrés por el trabajo.

La Dra. Soto asintió y comenzó con el procedimiento de rutina: le tomó la presión, escuchó su corazón y sus pulmones. Todo parecía normal.

—Muy bien, ahora voy a examinarte el abdomen y la espalda. ¿Te puedes recostar, por favor?

Mientras Laura se recostaba, la manga de su blusa se deslizó ligeramente, revelando un **moretón** de un color amarillento y violáceo en la parte superior de su brazo, un lugar poco común para un golpe accidental. Laura se apresuró a bajar la manga, un gesto rápido y casi inconsciente.

La Dra. Soto lo notó, pero no dijo nada en ese momento. Continuó con el examen físico sin alterar su rutina, manteniendo una conversación ligera para que Laura no se sintiera bajo escrutinio. Sin embargo, su mente ya estaba trabajando, conectando la fatiga en los ojos de Laura, su mención al "estrés" y el moretón oculto.

Una vez que terminó el examen físico y Laura volvió a sentarse, la Dra. Soto cerró la puerta del consultorio, un pequeño gesto para asegurar la privacidad. Se sentó frente a ella, su tono cambió de clínico a genuinamente preocupado.

—Laura, todo en tu examen físico se ve bien. Pero noté un moretón en tu brazo. A veces, el estrés del que me hablas no solo viene del trabajo.

Hizo una pausa, creando un espacio seguro. —Voy a hacerte una pregunta que les hago a todas mis pacientes, porque su bienestar es mi prioridad número uno. ¿Te sientes segura en casa?

El aire en la habitación pareció detenerse. La pregunta, hecha con tanta calma y sin juicio, colgó entre ellas. Los ojos de Laura se llenaron de lágrimas que había estado conteniendo por mucho tiempo. Negó con la cabeza lentamente, una sola vez.

Ese simple gesto lo confirmó todo.

La Dra. Soto no presionó para obtener detalles. No preguntó "¿quién?" o "¿cómo?". Sabía que el primer paso no era interrogar, sino ofrecer apoyo incondicional.

—Gracias por tu valentía al responderme —dijo con voz suave—. No tienes que contarme nada que no quieras. Lo más importante es que sepas que no estás sola y que lo que está pasando no es tu culpa.

Abrió un cajón de su escritorio y sacó un pequeño folleto sin logotipos llamativos, diseñado para ser discreto.

—Existen **recursos** para ayudarte. Este folleto tiene un número de teléfono de una línea de ayuda local. Es confidencial y están disponibles 24 horas al día. Puedes llamar solo para hablar, para hacer un plan de **seguridad**, o para que te conecten con refugios y asesores legales si alguna vez lo necesitas.

Colocó el folleto boca abajo sobre la mesa, dándole a Laura el control de tomarlo o no.

—No tienes que hacer nada ahora. Solo quiero que tengas esta información. Puedes guardarla en un lugar seguro. Mi consultorio es un lugar seguro para ti, Laura. Siempre puedes venir aquí, incluso si solo necesitas un lugar donde estar tranquila por diez minutos.

Laura finalmente rompió el silencio, su voz apenas un susurro. —Tengo miedo.

—Lo sé —respondió la Dra. Soto, su voz llena de empatía—. El miedo es la herramienta más poderosa del abuso. Pero la información es la tuya. Y hoy has dado un paso muy valiente al reconocerlo.

Laura tomó el folleto y lo guardó en su bolso sin mirarlo. Cuando se levantó para irse, miró a la Dra. Soto a los ojos, y esta vez, había algo más que cansancio en su mirada: una diminuta chispa de esperanza. Había venido por un **chequeo general**, pero se fue con algo mucho más valioso: la confirmación de que no estaba sola y una puerta abierta hacia la **seguridad**.

## Análisis de la Situación y Puntos Clave

**Nota Profesional y Lingüística:** La detección de la **violencia doméstica** es una responsabilidad crucial de los profesionales de la salud, especialmente en atención primaria, donde los pacientes pueden sentirse más cómodos. La clave es la detección de señales sutiles y el uso de un enfoque de detección universal y no estigmatizante.

### Vocabulario Médico Utilizado:

- **Chequeo general (General check-up)**: A menudo, es la única razón por la que un paciente en una situación de abuso puede tener para visitar a un médico, lo que convierte estas citas en oportunidades críticas para la intervención.

- ⊙ **Moretón (Bruise)**: El signo físico clave. La ubicación (en áreas generalmente cubiertas por la ropa) y el intento del paciente por ocultarlo son señales de alarma.

- ⊙ **Seguridad (Safety)**: La palabra central en la pregunta de detección. Preguntar sobre la "seguridad" es menos directo y acusatorio que preguntar sobre "abuso" o "violencia".

- ⊙ **Violencia doméstica (Domestic violence)**: El diagnóstico social subyacente.

- ⊙ **Recursos (Resources)**: El núcleo de la intervención. El rol del médico no es resolver el problema, sino conectar al paciente con los expertos y sistemas de apoyo que pueden hacerlo.

## Estrategia de Comunicación:

1. **Creación de un Entorno Seguro:** La Dra. Soto notó el signo físico pero esperó a estar en un momento privado y seguro (puerta cerrada, sentada frente a la paciente) para abordar el tema.

2. **Normalización de la Pregunta:** La frase "Esta es una pregunta que les hago a todas mis pacientes" es una técnica de detección universal recomendada. Reduce el estigma y la sensación de que la paciente está siendo señalada, lo que facilita una respuesta honesta.

3. **Enfoque en la Validación, no en la Investigación:** Una vez que Laura confirmó el problema, la doctora no pidió detalles del abuso. Esto es fundamental. El objetivo inmediato es validar los sentimientos de la víctima y ofrecer apoyo, no recopilar una historia detallada que podría ser traumática de contar.

4. **Provisión de Recursos Discretos:** El folleto sin marcas y la forma en que se lo ofreció (boca abajo, dándole el control a la paciente) respeta la necesidad de discreción y la autonomía de la víctima.

5. **Ofrecer Apoyo Concreto e Inmediato:** La oferta de que el consultorio es un "lugar seguro" es una intervención poderosa. Proporciona un refugio tangible e inmediato, aunque sea temporal.

6. **Empoderamiento a través de la Información:** La Dra. Soto enmarcó la situación como una lucha de poder: "El miedo es la herramienta del abuso. Pero la información es la tuya". Esto ayuda a la paciente a ver que tiene opciones y poder, lo cual es el primer paso para romper el ciclo de la violencia.

# "QUE DIOS LA BENDIGA, DOCTORA"

## La gratitud y la fe en la comunicación sobre cuidados paliativos

La Dra. Evans, una joven **oncóloga**, respiró hondo antes de entrar en la habitación. Dentro, la esperaba la familia de la señora Isabel, una mujer de 78 años con un cáncer de pulmón que había dejado de responder al tratamiento. La quimioterapia, que una vez fue una herramienta de esperanza, se había convertido en una fuente de sufrimiento.

En la habitación, el aire estaba cargado de una mezcla de amor y temor. El hijo de Isabel, Miguel, sostenía la mano de su madre. Su hija, Elena, estaba de pie junto a la ventana, mirando hacia afuera sin ver nada.

—Buenos días —dijo la Dra. Evans con voz suave, dirigiéndose a todos—. ¿Cómo ha pasado la noche la señora Isabel?

—No muy bien, doctora —respondió Miguel, sin soltar la mano de su madre—. La **tos** no la deja descansar y el dolor... el dolor es fuerte.

La Dra. Evans asintió. Había llegado el momento de tener la conversación más difícil en medicina, una que nunca se volvía más fácil.

—He revisado los últimos estudios y los resultados del tratamiento —comenzó, sentándose para estar al mismo nivel que ellos—. La quimioterapia ya no está funcionando como esperábamos. El cáncer sigue avanzando.

Hizo una pausa, permitiendo que el peso de sus palabras se asentara. —Hemos llegado a un punto en el que continuar con el tratamiento curativo le causaría a su madre más sufrimiento que beneficio.

Elena se giró, sus ojos llenos de lágrimas y un destello de lucha. —¿Quiere decir que se rinde? Mi madre es una luchadora. Siempre nos enseñó a tener **fe**.

La palabra **fe** era la clave. La Dra. Evans sabía que no podía hablar solo de medicina; tenía que hablar el lenguaje del corazón.

—No nos estamos rindiendo, Elena. De ninguna manera —respondió la doctora con una calidez firme—. Estamos cambiando el enfoque de la lucha. Ya no luchamos contra la enfermedad, porque esa batalla se ha vuelto demasiado dura para el cuerpo de su madre. Ahora, vamos a luchar por ella. Vamos a luchar por su **calidad de vida**.

Se inclinó hacia la señora Isabel, que la miraba con ojos cansados pero lúcidos. —¿Isabel, qué es lo más importante para usted en este momento?

La anciana tardó en responder, su voz un susurro. —No tener dolor. Y estar con ellos.

—Exactamente —dijo la Dra. Evans, validando sus deseos—. Y ese es nuestro nuevo plan. Vamos a enfocar todos nuestros esfuerzos en el **manejo del dolor** y en su **confort**. Queremos que sus días sean tranquilos, que pueda hablar con su familia, que esté en paz. A esto lo llamamos **cuidados paliativos**.

Miguel la miró, con una pregunta en los ojos. —¿Eso significa que la mandamos a casa a morir?

—Significa que la cuidamos intensamente, pero con un objetivo diferente —aclaró la doctora—. El objetivo ya no es la cura, sino el bienestar. Podemos manejar el dolor con medicamentos más fuertes. Tenemos enfermeras, trabajadores sociales, incluso un capellán si lo desean, todo un equipo para apoyarlos a ustedes y a ella. La meta es que cada día que le quede, sea un buen día.

Elena, que había estado llorando en silencio, se acercó a la cama. Miró a su madre y luego a la doctora. —Mi mamá siempre dice que todo está en manos de Dios.

—Y yo respeto profundamente esa **fe** —respondió la Dra. Evans—. La medicina tiene sus límites, y es aquí donde la fe y el amor toman el papel más importante. Mi trabajo es asegurarme de que el camino de su madre sea lo más suave y digno posible, mientras ustedes la acompañan con su amor y su fe.

La conversación duró casi una hora. Hablaron de los miedos, de los deseos, de los detalles prácticos. Al final, un sentido de calma había reemplazado la tensión inicial. No era resignación, sino aceptación.

Al despedirse, Elena le tomó la mano a la Dra. Evans. —Gracias, doctora. Nadie nos lo había explicado así. Nos ha dado paz.

Miguel asintió, con los ojos enrojecidos. —Que Dios la bendiga, doctora.

La Dra. Evans salió de la habitación con una mezcla de humildad y propósito. En oncología, las victorias no siempre eran curas. A veces, la victoria más grande era una conversación honesta, un dolor aliviado, y una familia que podía encontrar paz en medio de la despedida, sostenida por la medicina, el amor y la fe.

## Análisis de la Situación y Puntos Clave

**Nota Profesional y Lingüística:** Las conversaciones sobre el final de la vida son de las más desafiantes. Requieren una combinación de honestidad clínica, empatía profunda y respeto por las creencias espirituales y culturales del paciente y su familia. La **fe** es a menudo un pilar central para las familias hispanas, y debe ser integrada en la conversación, no vista como un obstáculo para la aceptación médica.

## Vocabulario Médico Utilizado:

- ⊙ **Oncóloga (Oncologist):** La especialista que trata el cáncer.
- ⊙ **Tratamiento curativo (Curative treatment):** El enfoque médico que busca curar la enfermedad. Es importante diferenciarlo del tratamiento paliativo.
- ⊙ **Calidad de vida / Confort (Quality of life / Comfort):** Los nuevos objetivos del cuidado cuando la cura ya no es posible.
- ⊙ **Manejo del dolor (Pain management):** Una de las principales prioridades en los cuidados paliativos.
- ⊙ **Cuidados paliativos (Palliative care):** El enfoque de atención integral que se centra en el confort y la calidad de vida. Es crucial explicar que no significa "abandonar" al paciente.
- ⊙ **Fe (Faith):** El concepto cultural y espiritual que guía la perspectiva de la familia y que la doctora debe respetar e integrar.

## Estrategia de Comunicación:

1. **Establecer un Tono Empático:** La Dra. Evans comenzó la conversación con calma, sentándose y mostrando que tenía tiempo para ellos, lo que indicó que era una discusión importante y no apresurada.

2. **Honestidad con Compasión:** Fue directa sobre el **pronóstico** y la ineficacia del tratamiento, pero lo hizo con un lenguaje suave y compasivo, evitando términos clínicos duros.

3. **Reencuadrar el Objetivo:** La estrategia más poderosa fue cambiar el paradigma de "rendirse" a "cambiar el enfoque de la lucha". Esto permitió a la familia, especialmente a Elena, seguir sintiendo que estaban haciendo algo activo y amoroso por su madre.

4. **Involucrar al Paciente:** A pesar de su debilidad, la doctora se dirigió directamente a la señora Isabel para preguntarle por sus deseos. Esto centró la conversación en la autonomía y la dignidad del paciente.

5. **Integrar la Fe en la Conversación:** En lugar de ver la fe como una barrera para la toma de decisiones médicas, la Dra. Evans la validó y la posicionó como un recurso de fortaleza para la familia, trabajando en paralelo con el cuidado médico.

6. **Definir Claramente los Cuidados Paliativos:** Explicó que los **cuidados paliativos** son una forma activa e intensa de cuidado, no un abandono. Aclaró el rol del equipo multidisciplinario, lo que proporcionó a la familia una sensación de apoyo integral.

# GLOSSARY OF COMMON MEDICAL TERMS (ENGLISH – SPANISH)[4]

This glossary is adapted from internationally accepted terminology systems, including MeSH (Medical Subject Headings, NLM), ICD-10 (WHO), and PAHO/WHO terminology guidelines.

Sources:

- ⊙ MeSH: https://meshb.nlm.nih.gov
- ⊙ ICD-10: https://icd.who.int/browse10/2019/en
- ⊙ PAHO/WHO: https://iris.paho.org/handle/10665.2/52150

**Administrative**

| English | Spanish |
| --- | --- |
| Address | Dirección |
| Appointment | Cita |
| Attending physician | Médico de turno |
| Child | Niño/Niña |
| Clinic | Clínica |
| Clinical record | Historia Clínica |
| Date of birth | Fecha de nacimiento |
| Doctor / physician | Médico / Médica |
| Emergency | Emergencia |
| Emergency room | Urgencias / Sala de emergencias |
| Family | Familia |
| Follow-up appointment | Cita de seguimiento / Cita de control |

| English | Spanish |
|---------|---------|
| Full name | Nombre completo |
| Gastroenterology | Gastroenterología |
| Healthcare professionals | Profesionales de la salud |
| Hospital | Hospital |
| Hospitalization | Hospitalización |
| Insurance | Seguro médico |
| Last name | Apellido |
| Medical appointments | Citas médicas |
| Medical history | Historial médico |
| Medical interpreter | Intérprete médico |
| Name | Nombre |
| Nurse | Enfermero / Enfermera |
| Patient | Paciente |
| Pharmacy | Farmacia |
| Phone number | Número de teléfono |
| Physical therapy | Fisioterapia / Terapia física |
| Procedure | Procedimiento |
| Radiology technician | Técnico de radiología |
| Rehabilitation | Rehabilitación |
| Surgery | Cirugía |

## Alternative and Supportive Therapies

| English | Spanish |
|---------|---------|
| Alternative treatments | Tratamientos alternativos |
| Therapy | Terapia |

## Anatomy

| English | Spanish |
| --- | --- |
| Abdomen | Abdomen |
| Arm | Brazo |
| Back | Espalda |
| Blood | Sangre |
| Body | Cuerpo |
| Bone | Hueso |
| Brain | Cerebro |
| Chest | Pecho |
| Colon | Colon |
| Ear | Oído |
| Eye | Ojo |
| Finger | Dedos de las manos |
| Foot | Pie |
| Hand | Mano |
| Head | Cabeza |
| Heart | Corazón |
| Kidney | Riñón |
| Knee | Rodilla |
| Leg | Pierna |
| Limbs | Extremidades |
| Liver | Hígado |
| Lower back | Zona lumbar |
| Lung | Pulmón |
| Muscle | Músculo |
| Nerve | Nervio |

| English | Spanish |
| --- | --- |
| Organ | Órgano |
| Ovary | Ovario |
| Prostate | Próstata |
| Skin | Piel |
| Stomach | Estómago |
| Testicle | Testículo |
| Throat | Garganta |
| Thyroid | Tiroides |
| Toes | Dedos de los pies |
| Urine | Orina |
| Uterus | Útero |
| Vein | Vena |

## Common Diseases and Conditions

| English | Spanish |
| --- | --- |
| Alcohol use disorder / Alcohol abuse | Alcoholismo |
| Allergy | Alergia |
| Anemia | Anemia |
| Blood pressure | Presión arterial / Tensión arterial |
| Cancer | Cáncer |
| Cardiovascular disease | Enfermedad cardiovascular |
| Chronic illnesses / chronic conditions | Enfermedades crónicas |
| Cold | Resfriado |
| Condition / illness / disease | Condición / enfermedad |
| Diabetes | Diabetes |
| Emotional support | Apoyo emocional |

| English | Spanish |
|---|---|
| Fracture | Fractura |
| Genetic predisposition | Predisposición genética |
| Health | Salud |
| High Blood Pressure | Hipertensión / Presión alta |
| Hypertension / High blood pressure | Hipertensión |
| Measles | Sarampión |
| Migraine | Migraña |
| Palliative care | Cuidados paliativos |
| Pregnancy | Embarazo |
| Pregnant | Embarazada |
| Stroke | Derrame cerebral / Accidente cerebrovascular (ACV) |
| Tumor | Tumor |
| Varicella (chickenpox) | Varicela |
| Wound | Herida |

## Diagnostics and Tests

| English | Spanish |
|---|---|
| CT scan | Tomografía computarizada |
| Diagnosis | Diagnóstico |
| ECG (Electrocardiogram) | Electrocardiograma |
| Echocardiogram | Ecocardiograma |
| Endoscopy | Endoscopia |
| Glucose | Glucosa |
| MRI (Magnetic Resonance Imaging) | Resonancia magnética |
| Pap smear | Papanicolaou / Citología vaginal o cervical |
| Ultrasound | Ultrasonido / Ecografía |
| X-ray | Radiografía |

## Medical Equipment and Supplies

| English | Spanish |
| --- | --- |
| Gloves | Guantes |
| Otoscope | Otoscopio |
| Reflex hammer | Martillo de reflejos |
| Stethoscope | Estetoscopio |

## Medications and Drug Use

| English | Spanish |
| --- | --- |
| Dose | Dosis |
| Drug | Droga / Medicamento |
| Frequency (of use) | Frecuencia (de uso) |
| Injection | Inyección |
| Insulin | Insulina |
| Intravenous (IV) | Intravenosa / endovenosa |
| Illicit substances | Substancia ilegales |
| Medication | Medicamento / Medicación |
| Medication / Drug | Medicamento / Fármaco |
| Oral (administration) | Vía oral |
| Over-the-counter (OTC) | Sin receta / De venta libre |
| Prescription | Receta |
| Recreational drugs | Drogas ilegales |
| Sedation | Sedación |
| Side effect | Efecto secundario |

## Physical Examination

| English | Spanish |
| --- | --- |
| Auscultation | Auscultación |
| Bend / Flex | Doblar / Flexionar |
| Breath | Respiración |
| Check / assess reflexes | Revisar / evaluar los reflejos |
| Examination | Examen / Revisión |
| Heart rate | Frecuencia cardíaca |
| Lie on your back | Acostarse boca arriba |
| Oxygen level | Nivel de oxígeno |
| Pain scale | Escala del dolor |
| Palpation | Palpación |
| Percussion | Percusión |
| Pressure | Presión |
| Pulse | Pulso |
| Respiratory rate | Frecuencia respiratoria |
| Temperature | Temperatura |
| Vital signs | Signos vitales |

## Signs and Symptoms

| English | Spanish |
| --- | --- |
| Abdominal pain | Dolor abdominal |
| Associated symptoms | Síntomas asociados |
| Asthma | Asma |
| Breathing difficulty | Dificultad para respirar |
| Chills | Escalofríos |

| English | Spanish |
|---------|---------|
| Constipation | Estreñimiento / Constipación |
| Contraction | Contracción |
| Cough | Tos |
| Cramp | Calambre |
| Deep | Profundo |
| Dementia | Demencia |
| Diarrhea | Diarrea |
| Discomfort | Molestia |
| Dizziness | Mareo |
| Fatigue | Fatiga |
| Fever | Fiebre |
| Flu | Gripe |
| Headaches | Dolores de cabeza |
| Hold your breath | Mantener el aire |
| Infection | Infección |
| Inflammation | Inflamación |
| Loss of appetite | Pérdida de apetito |
| Nausea | Náusea |
| Night sweats | Sudoración nocturna |
| Pain | Dolor |
| Pain / Discomfort | Dolor / Molestia |
| Rash | Erupción |
| Relax your muscles | Relajar los músculos |
| Sensitive | Sensible |

| English | Spanish |
| --- | --- |
| Sharp pain | Dolor punzante |
| Sore throat | Dolor de garganta |
| Stabbing pain | Punzada |
| Symptom | Síntoma |
| Vomiting | Vómito |
| Waiting room | Sala de espera |
| Worsen the pain | Empeorar el dolor |

## Vaccination and Prevention

| English | Spanish |
| --- | --- |
| Relieve the pain | Aliviar el dolor |
| Treatment | Tratamiento |
| Vaccine | Vacuna |

# COMMON SPANISH PHRASES FOR PATIENT INTERACTIONS

Effective communication during patient encounters is essential for delivering high-quality care to Spanish-speaking patients. This appendix offers healthcare providers a practical, quick-reference list of commonly used Spanish phrases that can be integrated into routine clinical practice. Using these phrases helps establish trust, reduce patient anxiety, and ensure accurate understanding throughout the medical encounter.

Quick-Reference Phrases for Clinical Encounters:

- *¿Cómo se siente hoy?* — How are you feeling today?
- *¿Dónde le duele?* — Where does it hurt?
- *Respire profundo.* — Take a deep breath.
- *Vamos a hacer un examen físico.* — We're going to do a physical exam.
- *¿Está tomando algún medicamento?* — Are you taking any medication?
- *Regrese en dos semanas para una cita de seguimiento.* — Come back in two weeks for a follow-up appointment.
- *Le voy a tomar la presión arterial.* — I'm going to take your blood pressure.
- *Abra la boca.* — Open your mouth.
- *Necesito que se quite la ropa hasta la cintura.* — I need you to undress to the waist.
- *Por favor, acuéstese boca arriba.* — Please lie on your back.
- *Avíseme si siente dolor.* — Let me know if you feel pain.
- *No se preocupe.* — Don't worry.
- *Voy a explicarle los resultados.* — I will explain the results to you.
- *Es importante que tome este medicamento.* — It's important that you take this medication.
- *Si tiene preguntas, no dude en preguntar.* — If you have questions, don't hesitate to ask.
- *Cuídese mucho.* — Take good safe care of yourself.

**Best Practices for Using Spanish Phrases in Patient Care**

- Speak slowly and clearly to ensure patient understanding.
- Use appropriate tone and body language to convey empathy and respect.
- Always verify comprehension, especially when giving instructions.
- When in doubt, use professional medical interpreters for complex discussions.
- Practice regularly to build confidence and fluency in clinical conversations.

# BIBLIOGRAPHY

**1  Cultural Note on the Use of the Term "Drug"**

National Institute on Drug Abuse. (2022). *Your Words Matter – Language Showing Compassion and Care for Women, Infants, Families, and Communities Impacted by Substance Use Disorder.* NIDAMED. Retrieved from https://nida.nih.gov/nidamed-medical-health-professionals/health-professions-education/words-matter-language-showing-compassion-care-women-infants-families-communities-impacted-substance-use-disorder

Pan American Health Organization. (2021, December 27). PAHO launches project to improve policies on substance use disorders [*Lanzamiento de un proyecto para mejorar políticas sobre trastornos por uso de sustancias*]. OPS/PAHO. Retrieved from https://www.paho.org

**2  Cultural Note about the Use of "Don" and "Doña":**

Boricuagenes. (s. f.). *Genealogical use of Don & Doña*. Retrieved from https://boricuagenes.com/genealogical-use-of-don-dona/

Folan, W. J. (1967). *Don and doñaship terminology in Merida, Yucatan, Mexico. América Indígena*, 27(1). Retrieved from https://es.scribd.com/document/663043175/Don-and-donaship-terminology-in-Merida-Yucatan-Mexico-Folan-W-J

Spanish Academy Antigüena. (s. f.). Don - *Honorific title explained and how to use it*. Recuperado de https://www.spanishacademyantiguena.com/blog/2018/11/05/don-honorific-title-explained-and-how-to-use-it/

El País (Colombia): Herrera, J. S. (2018, enero). *¿Por qué los colombianos decimos don y doña? El País Cali*. Retrieved from https://www.elpais.com.co/entretenimiento/cultura/por-que-los-colombianos-decimos-don-y-dona.html

**3  Visual Analogue Scale (VAS)**

Delgado, D. A., Lambert, B. S., Boutris, N., McCulloch, P. C., Robbins, A. B., Moreno, M. R., & Harris, J. D. (2018). Validation of digital visual analog scale pain scoring with a traditional paper-based visual analog scale in adults. Journal of the American Academy of Orthopaedic Surgeons Global Research & Reviews, 2(3), e088. https://doi.org/10.5435/JAAOSGlobal-D-17-0008

Pardo, C., Muñoz, T., Chamorro, C., & Analgesia and Sedation Work Group of SEMICYUC. (2006). Monitoring pain: Recommendations of the Analgesia and Sedation Work Group of

SEMICYUC. Medicina Intensiva, 30(8), 387–400. https://scielo.isciii.es/scielo.php?script=sci_arttext&pid=S0210-56912006000800004

**4 Medical Spanish Vocabulary Resources for English Speakers**

Poliglota. (2022, 3 de junio). *Vocabulario médico en inglés: Conoce las palabras más usadas.* Retrieved from: https://www.poliglota.org/post/vocabulario-medico-en-ingles

don Quijote. (s.f.). *Vocabulario médico en español.* Retrieved from: https://www.donquijote.org/es/blog/vocabulario-medico/

Sprachcaffe. (s.f.). *Vocabulario médico en español.* Retrieved from: https://www.sprachcaffe.com/espanol/cursos-espanol-extranjero/aprende-espanol/vocabulario-espanol/vocabulario-para-niveles-intermedios-espanol/vocabulario-medico-espanol.htm

## APPENDIX D

# BOOKS BY THIS AUTHOR

If you enjoyed this book and want to keep improving your Spanish through fun and engaging reading, don't miss my other bestselling collections:

**80 Short Stories in Spanish – Volume 1**

A unique mix of beginner to advanced stories designed to expand your vocabulary and boost your confidence step by step.

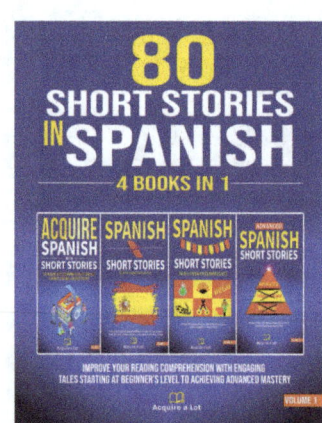

**80 Spanish Short Stories – Volume 2**

A brand-new collection of fresh stories that will challenge and entertain you while helping you achieve fluency.

Both volumes are perfect for learners of all levels, featuring questions, answers, and vocabulary lists to make learning practical and enjoyable.

**Find them on Amazon by searching for the titles.**

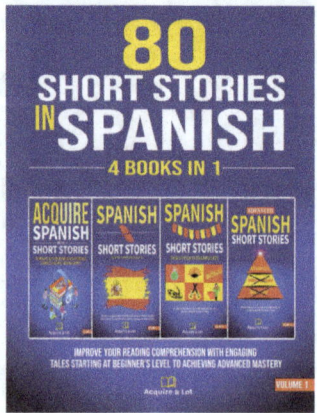

www.ingramcontent.com/pod-product-compliance
Lightning Source LLC
Chambersburg PA
CBHW080818120626
46556CB00010B/3324